Breaking Free from Long Covid

of related interest

Chronic Fatigue Syndrome/ME
Support for Family and Friends
Elizabeth Turp
ISBN 978 1 84905 141 5
eISBN 978 0 85700 347 8

Pain is Really Strange
Steve Haines
Illustrated by Sophie Standing
ISBN 978 1 84819 264 5
eISBN 978 0 85701 212 8
... is Really Strange series

Anxiety is Really Strange
Steve Haines
Illustrated by Sophie Standing
ISBN 978 1 84819 389 5
eISBN 978 0 85701 345 3
... is Really Strange series

Pulling Through
Help for Families Navigating Life-Changing Illness
Catherine Jessop
ISBN 978 1 78775 372 3
eISBN 978 1 78775 373 0

BREAKING FREE
from
LONG COVID

*Reclaiming Life and the
Things that Matter*

Dr Lucy Gahan

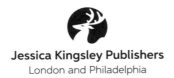

Jessica Kingsley Publishers
London and Philadelphia

First published in Great Britain in 2023 by Jessica Kingsley Publishers
An imprint of Hodder & Stoughton Ltd
An Hachette Company

1

A CIP catalogue record for this title is available from the
British Library and the Library of Congress

ISBN 978 1 83997 350 5
eISBN 978 1 83997 351 2

Printed and bound in Great Britain by TJ Books Ltd

Jessica Kingsley Publishers' policy is to use papers that are natural,
renewable and recyclable products and made from wood grown in
sustainable forests. The logging and manufacturing processes are expected
to conform to the environmental regulations of the country of origin.

Jessica Kingsley Publishers
Carmelite House
50 Victoria Embankment
London EC4Y 0DZ

www.jkp.com

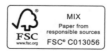

MIX
Paper from
responsible sources
FSC
www.fsc.org
FSC® C013056

*For every person who lives each day with invisible illness
and to those who believe us.*
To B, E and N, for keeping me close to what matters most.

Contents

Acknowledgements

Elizabeth Gilbert, in her book *Big Magic* (2016), presents ideas as forms of magic, swirling around us, looking for willing human partners to bring them into being. The idea for this book seemed to visit me when I was barely able to get out of bed in summer 2020, a whisper that said 'this *has* to be talked about more'. Despite my fragile physical state, I felt driven to share not only my story of Long Covid, but all the things I was learning from others who were helping me to make sense of what was happening to me. This book is not only my story, but also a drawing together of ideas, theories, concepts, hypotheses and stories from people from all different walks of life. It is a sharing of the key ideas which helped me get through the darkest times of Long Covid. Each one of you who has been with me through this experience, or who has taught me something, has contributed in ways which are beyond description or measure.

This book would not have been possible without the community of people with Long Covid across the world who have contributed to the Long Haul Covid Fighters Facebook group. Your sharing of stories and discoveries has accompanied me and so many others through the most frightening of experiences. I would not have made any of the connections, learnings and discoveries without you. Thank you, Amy Watson, Kate Porter and Ashley F for your tireless hard work in setting up and maintaining the group despite your own health struggles. Your work makes a crucial difference to so many.

So much of what we are learning about Long Covid is only there because of who has gone before us. We are not the first people to have the authenticity of our symptoms doubted. I would like to acknowledge everyone who bears the burden of illness which is invisible to others or doubted in some way, and who continually has to work to be seen and acknowledged.

Those who do validate our experiences, whether in a personal or a professional context, make a crucial difference. A special thank you to Dr Bale for being one of the first professionals who did that for me, bringing validation and meaning to what looked like the ordinary.

A special thank you to Hugh Fox, my mentor and 'co-conspirator'! Thank you for giving your time freely to accompany me from the very beginning when I said to you that I didn't dare write a book but I seemed to be doing it anyway! Each of our conversations has left me inspired, focused and energised, with a little bit more knowledge about how to go forward.

To Sarah Hamlin, Maddy Budd, Carys Homer and everyone at Jessica Kingsley Publishers. When I started putting words on paper I didn't know how I was going to get them 'out there' to share with the people I most wanted to. You make visible the stories that don't necessarily get told elsewhere. Thank you for giving me that chance, and for doing it with such care. A special thank you to Kara McHale for a beautiful cover.

Kaethe Weingarten – well before Long Covid came along, your work on narratives of illness has been a major influence on my conversations with people going through serious illness. It then accompanied me at a time when I most needed to make some sense of the turmoil of my own illness, and I desperately wanted to share some of it with other people going through Long Covid. Thank you for allowing me to do this here. In a training course I once attended, you talked about there always being 'wiggle room', even in the most difficult of circumstances, and this has always stayed with me.

Noah Greenspan – your Pulmonary Wellness Foundation video describing dysautonomia was a turning point for me, validating and making sense of what seemed like a bizarre set of symptoms. Your videos helped me through the worst of my Long Covid journey and I'm so thankful for your ongoing work to not only make Long Covid visible, but to find answers and ways through.

David Denborough, thank you for allowing me to share ideas and concepts from your book *Retelling the Stories of Our Lives* (2014), particularly the Team of Life, which has inspired me to construct my own 'virtual team' in response to Long Covid.

Thank you to everyone at the Physical Health Psychology Team in which I've worked for the last ten years. Thank you especially to Heidi for your trust, kindness and always seeming to value whatever I've had to offer.

Thank you to Kevin Manley and Kath Raymond Hinton for your early advice about contracts and to Josh Duntz, Noah Greenspan, Llinos Llafar Rollinson and Alice Riley for reading early copies of the book.

Thank you to my family and friends who have been with me through the last two years, and who have each in your own ways helped me to remember the me that is not Long Covid.

Mum and Tony, for your encouragement, for building railways, playing chess and entertaining the boys so I could 'get on'! Mum, thank you for showing me the importance of speaking out and questioning the taken-for-granted, and demonstrating that you don't need to be an extrovert to take some action.

Dad, you were never afraid to say or do something different to everyone else if it felt important enough. Thank you for teaching me to think for myself, whilst also being the kindest and most gentle person I've ever met.

Thank you to Caroline, my wonderful sister, for being my most enthusiastic supporter, for trying to promote this book before it was even finished and for sending me an oximeter before I even knew what one was!

Nana and Grandad – I have always admired your thirst for knowledge and education. You always showed genuine interest in what I was learning. Although you didn't quite get to read this, I know you'd be proud.

Helen, thank you for attentively and tirelessly talking with me about Long Covid nearly every Friday(!), and for seeing that what mattered wasn't just in the publishing but in the taking of some action. Thank you to you and Martin for feeding and entertaining the boys so that I could be writing!

Marilyn, it's such a privilege to have you as my friend. Thank you for just 'getting it' and for laughing with me through it all!

Thank you, Vivien, for your quiet wisdom through many years of friendship and for being one of the most acknowledging people I could ever meet.

Thank you, Llinos, for helping me at a distance through 'round one' and for being the person to whom I don't need to explain!

Thank you, John and Margaret, for the early food parcels!

For all the people on my 'Team' – those who hopefully do know it – Kate, Monika, Sarah, Paul and Marie, and those who don't, but who, without even knowing it, help me each day – Yoga with Adriene and the Stasis Post Covid Programme.

And of course, to E, B and N – the reason for it all.

Introduction

'Covid only lasts two weeks.' The doctor shakes her head slowly. I search her face for something more, a clue as to what's going to happen next, but I can't find anything, she gives nothing away. But she's not launching into action. I'm confused, not sure what to make of it, but it doesn't feel right. Apparently, my ECG and blood tests are 'normal'. But that can't be it. The beta blocker which my GP gave me yesterday has calmed my heart a little, but my whole body is still shaky and wobbly with the most frightening sensation in my chest. I'm not sure if it feels as though an elephant is sitting on it or is going to burst out of it. The doctor seems to tower over me. I can see that she's not particularly tall, but I feel small and quite pathetic, slumped on the hospital trolley with my mask stretched across my face. I'd been terrified of coming to A&E, fearing they'd whisk me off somewhere and not let me out, that I wouldn't be able to see my children. But the storm inside my body became too much, and when I got here the wave of relief that I'm no longer on my own with this took over. I was sure they'd sort out whatever was happening to me. The doctor murmurs something about staying away from things which make me anxious, like the Facebook group I'd mentioned. The one thing which has been keeping me sane, telling me that I'm not the only one

going through this hell. The hope I held onto drops out of the bottom of my stomach and I feel slightly sick. She doesn't believe me. She think I'm anxious, too anxious. Her face gives it away. I know my chance has gone. I can't find the words to form an intelligent, considered response so I mumble 'I'm a clinical psychologist and I'm not anxious!' but it sounds quiet and small and slightly desperate. I just need to get out of here. I'm on my own with this.

This was me in May 2020, a few weeks after I thought I'd recovered from Covid. It seems like it happened years ago, to another version of me, in a different time. Long Covid has taken all that I took for granted as being stable in my life, lifted it up, shaken it, put it down again and left me to make sense of what was left, like one of those snow globes, except not so pretty. How could this have happened to me? I must have taken a wrong turn and stepped into a story that just wasn't meant for me. If you have Long Covid you'll know – you'll know that what happened to me on that day in the hospital wasn't unique or special – it could have been written by tens of thousands of people with Long Covid, and it may have happened to you. Having my body taken over by a sinister presence which seemed invisible to the people whose help I most needed has been just one of many challenges that is living with Long Covid.

From that day in A&E, I felt that I was on my own; that I was going to have to figure out for myself how to get out of this, whatever 'this' was. I wasn't a medical doctor, and I didn't have a clue what I was going to do, I just knew that I felt more ill than I'd ever felt in my life, yet doctors didn't seem to see it. I had no grand plan of how I was going to sort this out. I could barely stand up! Having made it through the initial illness I was apparently supposed to recover within a couple of weeks.

But I was certain I wasn't imagining the symptoms – I'd joined a Facebook group with a rapidly growing number of people across the world who were all experiencing multiple weird and frightening symptoms, weeks after having Covid, which just weren't getting better. There was no way I was giving it up: it wasn't making me anxious; it was keeping me sane. I'd joined the thousands of other people who knew just how Long Covid can make you feel in your body – an individual yet collective experience of trying to figure out how to get answers to what was happening to us.

I wrote this book because of that time, when I felt completely lost. No one in the medical profession seemed to know how to help me yet I didn't know how to help myself either. The despair I felt that day in the hospital was just the beginning of the story. For weeks and months, I scanned the Facebook group for clues and answers, and every so often I'd stumble on something which seemed to make a difference to my symptoms. Each discovery sparked another connection and I gathered information, tricks, tools, ideas and theories about Long Covid like a magpie collecting precious little gems. I started to be able to respond; to take small actions rather than feeling entirely at the mercy of Long Covid. Yet the challenges weren't just physical. The longer it went on, the more disconnected I was becoming from my old life, from the things I could do before and who I thought I was. I became weary of trying to explain to people that no, I'm still not better. I remembered some of Kaethe Weingarten's writing about narratives of illness. I'd drawn on these ideas so many times in my conversations at work with people going through serious illness, but now they were taking on a new life. My feelings of fear, anger, isolation and a sense of people just not 'getting it' made sense. As I read more and more stories from the Long Covid forums, it became clear that I wasn't alone in these struggles, many of which seemed invisible to the outside world. Surely if I'd found these ideas helpful, then I should find a way of sharing them?

At that time writing a book wasn't something that I could ever imagine doing. I'd sit in bed on beautiful sunny days in June 2020 and hear the shrieks and chatter of my children going for walks with my partner – the same walks we did together just a few weeks earlier. I was barely able to get to the bathroom. I remember thinking, 'If I can go for a walk again, I'll have made it. I'll be happy.' I'm not a writer; I wasn't even sure I could make any sense of what was in my head, let alone put it down on paper. But perhaps no one's a writer until they've got something to say. And I couldn't keep quiet. The only people talking about Long Covid seemed to be the people who had it – to the rest of the world we seemed barely visible. Long Covid had done something to me, galvanised me into wanting to play a part, however small, in getting the real stories of Long Covid out there and talked about. It was at 100 days after my first Covid symptoms that I first had the urge to jot down some thoughts about what was happening to me. I called it '100 days of Covid'. It turned out that I was just having a 'good' day. After 20 minutes in front of my laptop I was back in bed, my heart racing. Months later when I tried again, I could barely concentrate for half an hour. Screens exhausted me and if I tried to write, my heart seemed to think I was running a marathon and the words I needed were frequently beyond my grasp. As months passed, I'd write a few lines, and then a few more, until I seemed to be writing a book. I didn't believe that I was capable, but I found myself doing it anyway. I'd made it this far and a 'why the hell not' attitude is one of the few side effects of Long Covid that I've welcomed.

My intentions in writing this book are two-fold. Most importantly, if your life has been turned upside down by Long

Covid, it is for you. From that first tentative moment of trying to put my thoughts on paper, it has been about reaching the person who might just be where I was, wondering if you'll ever be able to join in with the world again. I know our experiences will differ in ways, but I hope that you'll find something in these pages which resonates for you. Some of our symptoms might differ, but the thousands of posts I've read in Long Covid forums suggest that we share so many of the same challenges, some of which this book explores. I hope that the practical ideas will also contribute to you finding your own best ways to manage the challenges which Long Covid can bring about.

This book is also about making visible the real effects of Long Covid on people and their lives. Although Long Covid is increasingly being recognised as an illness, it is still often ignored, pushed aside or invalidated in the media, in the language used in relation to it and in decisions made by the Government in response to Covid. We are, of course, not the first people to experience this. People with illnesses or pain which is not necessarily visible or measurable in current medical tests have faced scepticism, disbelief and invalidation for decades. Those with chronic illnesses including ME/CFS (myalgic encephalomyelitis/chronic fatigue syndrome) and fibromyalgia, among others, have worked persistently to have their experiences validated and taken seriously. For me, Long Covid hasn't been about 'lingering' after-effects from Covid, as it is so often described in the media, but more like a tornado living inside my body, or as David Hare described Covid in his play Beat the Devil (2021) like having a 'dirty bomb thrown into your system'. The real, life-changing, often very frightening effects of Long Covid need to be seen, recognised and taken seriously. I know what it's like not to be seen, to have your experiences dismissed or minimised, adding to the distress of trying to navigate a new illness. Long Covid affects people's lives in every way imaginable – for me completely putting a halt to any meaningful functioning for well over a year. Twenty months later, and counting, despite now having a rich life in many ways, I still have to accommodate its effects. Other people are losing jobs, relationships and their previously healthy bodies – in other words, life as they knew it. The real stories of Long Covid need to be told so that Long Covid is taken seriously as a medical illness and people with Long Covid can get the medical, financial and social support we need. I hope that if you're reading this as a loved one of someone with Long Covid, or a professional working with people with Long Covid, that it helps you to understand better some of the challenges that people with Long Covid may be facing.

My intention in writing this book is to keep it as close as possible to my own experience, as an adult with Long Covid. I do not write here about Long Covid in children. However, I would like to explicitly acknowledge that longer-term effects of Long Covid are not limited to adults, and I have personal knowledge of ongoing Long Covid symptoms in children. Children must not be left behind in studying and treating Long Covid, nor should the effects of being parented by adults with Long Covid be ignored. There is an ongoing need for more research, and the narrative that children are by definition only mildly affected by Covid must be challenged.

I write this book both as a person with Long Covid and as a clinical psychologist and aspiring narrative therapist, both selves and perspectives woven throughout. My intention is not to present detailed theories from clinical psychology or narrative therapy, nor to offer advice or suggest that there is a 'right' way to manage Long Covid and its effects. We are all in unique positions in relation to Long Covid. Some people in the Long Covid forums consider themselves recovered. Others are still struggling with symptoms but able to get back to many of the things they used to do, and others are still in the midst of the most horrible and life-changing symptoms. This is a story of my experiences, many of which seem to have commonalities with the stories of so many people in Long Covid forums. It is about my thinking about, and making sense of, those experiences. Long Covid can take away so much of what matters to you. Many times I didn't believe that things would improve; that I'd ever have any quality of life again. During those times, I wanted someone to either tell me something I could do which might help me get through the day, or to give me some hope. So many people made a difference to me without even knowing it, including the people who have shared their experiences, ideas and stories in the Long Covid forums. Some of the ideas from narrative therapy have helped me to make sense of why the struggle of Long Covid can be so frightening and at times isolating, and have helped me to start to reclaim parts of my life which Long Covid has tried to take over. The ideas that I bring to you have sustained me and got me to where I am today. I hope I do them justice, that they contribute to your life as they have contributed to mine and give you some ideas about how to go forward.

The first half of the book explores some of the particular challenges of Long Covid, and how I moved from feeling unable to help myself to being able to take action and advocate for myself. I explore some of the effects of having an illness which can be so frightening and result in loss of parts of your life and yourself which matter so much, and how you might re-connect with some of the things which matter most to you. At the end of Chapter 7 is a worksheet in which I suggest you write down or talk through your responses. For me, it was the people with Long Covid in the online forums who could best understand what I was going through. Perhaps there may be scope for us to share our responses with each other.

The second half of the book is more practical. I explore some of the practices which have helped me most to manage my symptoms and helped me to regain a quality of life. If you've had Long Covid for any length of time you're likely to already have found many of your own strategies, but I hope this book will add to your own unique 'toolkit', in the way that other people have contributed to mine.

I've tried to make this book as 'brain-fog-accessible' as possible. I know it can be difficult to focus for any length of time, as I've found when trying to write it. It can be read from beginning to end, but you can also dip into it in any order. I've left space at the end of chapters for writing notes on anything you might want to remember or try to hold on to. At the end of some chapters are questions related to the contents of the chapter, to prompt further thinking if you want to and if they resonate with you in some way.

Throughout writing this book I have tried to hold in mind what it might be like to read someone's story with Long Covid when you are going through it yourself. I've wanted to write an honest and accurate account of what happened to me without glossing over the frightening details of my story. However, I also believe that it isn't always necessary to go into the distressing details in order to make sense of the effects and the responses we make (this fits with ways of working with trauma in narrative therapy which will be explored later in the book). Therefore, I have not gone into any unnecessary detail about particular events which may be distressing for people to read who may have gone through similar. I hope I have got this balance about right. The main narrative of my story and most of the detail of what happened to me is within Chapter I, and beyond this I focus more on themes and practical strategies.

In the writing of this book, I've had many moments of

doubt. Who am I to say anything about living through Long Covid? I think about people who are more seriously ill than me, who have lost a loved one to Covid and its effects, or who have lost their jobs or livelihood. What do I have to say to you? Can I possibly contribute in any way to what you've already survived so far? My hope is that this book is a contribution to a wider conversation and wealth of ideas, a piecing together of ways to minimise the devastating impact of Long Covid. Perhaps my contribution will only be small and only a tiny part of my story will resonate with you. It is at these times that I try to keep close the words of Kaethe Weingarten (2013b) in her work with people living through illness – that the small is not necessarily trivial. I hope that my story, and the ideas of those people who inspire me, will make a difference to you.

Chapter One

How It Started

I never thought I was at risk of serious effects of Covid. Perhaps I was too confident. I was in my early forties, healthy, only ever having had minor illnesses and fitter than I'd been for a long time. I wasn't blasé, but I was more concerned for other people in my life than I was for myself. Covid was creeping its way across the globe, and there were rumours of a lockdown heading our way, but the story was that you were mainly at risk if you were older or medically vulnerable. Even if I did catch it, it would apparently be no worse than a bad dose of flu. I'd taken up running in the last year, adding it to my regular routine of going to the gym. I had found a love of exercising and fitness since I was 21 when I discovered that, contrary to school PE experiences, I did in fact love exercise and movement, and trained as an exercise instructor while doing my degree. Since having children I'd also discovered yoga, which helped slow down my tendency to rush around from one thing to the next. Feeling fit and healthy made me feel, not indestructible, but that I didn't have to worry too much as I was probably in a good position to fight off a virus. I'd always been fascinated by the workings of the body and the mind – my first job in the NHS was working as a physiotherapy assistant in a neuro rehabilitation team where I learned a lot about working with both. Fast forward a few years and I had trained in clinical psychology and worked in both mental and physical health services. I thought I'd learned a lot about the relationship between the mind and body, but Covid was about to teach me more than I could ever have imagined.

In April 2020 I was more concerned about my partner or children getting Covid, assuming that if I caught it, I'd only be out of action for a couple of weeks. From where I am now, it's poignant and a bit eerie to see myself writing that. I envy that person who had such a sense of surety in her body.

For a few weeks I'd felt a bit under the weather. Throughout January 2020, roads had been closed due to flooding, and I'd been rushing around trying to keep up with school runs and driving over an hour each way to work. I was constantly running late and, bizarrely, I remember thinking that I just needed to slow down before I got ill. This was a few weeks before Covid.

It was 3rd April 2020 when I noticed that I couldn't take a full breath. I was in the car with my partner and two boys, collecting a vegetable box as we couldn't get a delivery. Although I was alarmed, it was such a vague feeling that I convinced myself I was either imagining it or having a panic attack. I'd never had a panic attack and wasn't sure why I'd have one now. Not wanting to alarm anyone I tried to conceal it. The feeling passed when I got out of the car and I didn't think any more of it. Two days later I just couldn't take a full breath. This time there was no convincing me it was anything other than Covid. You couldn't get tests at that time, but I didn't need one. I'd never felt anything like it.

This was the start of a frightening two weeks which passed in a blur of struggling to breathe punctuated by quieter times of just feeling too ill to get out of bed. Twenty-four hours later, my partner had the same symptoms. I don't know how we managed, but somehow we took turns to get up and do what was absolutely necessary to look after the boys. I remember sitting in bed trying to figure out how we could somehow, between us, make pasta for them! The boys spent unmentionable numbers of hours watching films and playing games on their iPad. We couldn't get food deliveries as the delivery slots were prioritised for the vulnerable, but we were lucky enough to have friends and family who dropped food parcels on our doorstep. I'm not sure what we would have done without them.

After two weeks we both seemed to be coming out the other side. For weeks it seemed to be wall-to-wall sunshine and I was spending hours sitting on our front lawn. We returned to our lockdown walks that we'd been taking before we got ill. We hadn't told family members who lived further away that we were ill as we hadn't wanted to worry them, but this seemed the right time to make the announcement – we'd had Covid and recovered!

Writing this feels like one of those 'Choose your own adventure' books you used to get free in cereal packets. This story could have gone two ways – what might have happened and what did happen. Our Covid story might have ended there, but it didn't.

It turns out that Covid is full of surprises. Not long after that announcement of recovery and seemingly out of nowhere, I became unable to stand up. If I tried, I'd feel lightheaded and have to sit down before I fell down. I started getting 'waves' of symptoms where my heart rate would inexplicably shoot up and my heart would beat with such ferocity that it felt as though it were trying to break out of my chest. I felt more ill than I'd ever felt. These waves would last a few hours before, inexplicably, a sense of equilibrium would return to my body. At this point I was having over 30 symptoms, including an unquenchable thirst and an internal tremor which other people couldn't see but was as though my whole body was shaking from the inside. I'd have sharp pains around my heart and, most terrifyingly, runs of arrhythmic heart beats which had me cowering in a foetal position on the sofa feeling that I was on the verge of having a heart attack. I had a bizarre feeling of fullness in my chest as though something was trying to burst out of it, a sensation which I could never explain to doctors but was possibly one of the worst feelings I had. I later found out that my blood pressure would either go sky high or drop like a stone when I moved positions. Strangely, though, in between these episodes, I'd be able to move around the house, though as a shadow of my usual self. I would force myself to look as normal as possible so as not to worry the boys too much, as if, somehow, they might not notice. On a 'good' day I'd take a few hours to slowly get dressed so that I could go along with my partner to pick up the children from school. Many times, just being upright in the car seemed to trigger the horrible feelings and I'd get through those seemingly endless car journeys through sheer stubborn willpower, just hanging on until I could crawl back up the stairs and into bed. I remember vividly having one 'episode' in the car where I knew my partner was talking to me, but I couldn't physically form words to respond to him. I still don't know what was happening in my body at this particular time, but it frightens me to think about it. I just had to get home.

You might wonder why I wasn't in hospital, or at least consulting a doctor? I was just too scared. The television was full of images of severely overcrowded hospitals crammed with people wearing what looked like spacesuits and rows of people on ventilators. I was convinced that if I went near a hospital my children wouldn't see me again, and if I contacted a GP, they might send me into hospital. When the waves took hold, I'd bargain with myself or I'd come to an agreement with my partner that if things didn't get better in one hour we'd call an ambulance, and time and again I'd ride through the symptoms and come out the other side.

At some point, this must have changed. I think I was so worn down by riding these bizarre waves of symptoms that I just wanted some help. Perhaps I'd gained a little confidence knowing that I'd made it through so far, and one day, with great trepidation I rang the Covid line. I was told that I'd rung the wrong line, I hadn't had Covid as I didn't have a cough or temperature. When I insisted the person on the line take a history of my symptoms, I eventually got to speak to an on-call GP. She had no answers for me but reassured me that I didn't need to go to hospital. The relief at having 'confessed' my symptoms to a medical professional and been told that I didn't need to go to hospital was overwhelming. I'd discovered the power of telling someone, sharing your fears. As a clinical psychologist I had a sense of the value of sharing emotional struggle, but I'd never experienced the intense relief that can come from sharing medical concerns.

This whole period of time is a blur of days and weeks which all merge into one, punctuated by events that stand out in my mind and don't seem to fit together into a coherent story. One day my symptoms would be calmer and I'd believe that this was it, I was finally getting better. Then something else would happen inside my body, seemingly out of the blue. One day my heart had been pounding hard and fast for hours and didn't seem to be letting up. It made me feel so ill and whatever I tried to calm it made no difference. I just couldn't take it anymore. Somehow my partner got me an in-surgery GP appointment, which were rare at this time due to risk of infection. Considering I could hardly stand up I don't know how I got to the appointment, but somehow I dressed and shuffled down the stairs. I'll never forget sitting at the bottom of the stairs looking out of the open front door at the ten steps across the grass to the car and wondering how on earth I'd make it. It seems that desperation can get you a long way, as somehow I made it across the lawn and eventually across the GP surgery where, with great relief, I found myself slumped against the wall in my GP's office, heart pounding, with the GP dressed like something from a dystopian film.

Long Covid has been described as a 'lucky dip' of symptoms, where you never know what you're going to get from one day to the next. The other random factor at play seems to be the care you get when you consult a medical professional with symptoms of Long Covid. That day, I hit the jackpot. It wouldn't have looked like anything extraordinary from the outside, but the way my GP got beside me, talked through my symptoms and problem-solved with me so that I could choose what to do next was not only practically incredibly helpful but emotionally just what I needed. She helped me to take action. I left with beta blockers to get me through the worst of the symptoms, and a plan to go to A&E the next day if things didn't improve. I spoke to this same GP every few weeks when new symptoms cropped up and each time we would talk through the symptoms and together, collaboratively, decide what to do next. It felt like great medical and psychological care in action and I decided there and then that if I get through this and I can have similar effects on people who consult with me then I will have done my job well.

The only predictable thing about the next few months was the unpredictability of each day. I'd take a few steps towards what looked like recovery, only to be suddenly interrupted by new symptoms, seemingly out of nowhere. This thing had a mind of its own. It felt just like the devil that David Hare described (2021), creeping through my body having its sinister way with a particular organ or system before going quiet, as though it were hiding out while deciding what to spring on me next. In October 2020 I spent around five weeks barely leaving the sofa as my oxygen levels would drop frighteningly low when I stood or even sat up. Throughout this my partner was trying to work at home as well as look after me and the children. Even on good days I could barely do anything at all. Most painful was wondering what would happen to me and how much my illness might be frightening my children. I'd save any scraps of energy to be with them at bedtime. I hated them seeing me ill in bed, so I'd put CBeebies stories on and lie next to them, crawling out of their beds only when they were asleep so that they didn't see me crawling out of their room. I got by in this barely functioning way for months. Sometimes I could get into the car and we'd drive to remote places in the countryside where the boys could play. I'd have my feet up on the dashboard to keep the blood from pooling in my legs and drink litres of coconut water for the electrolytes. Often, I'd feel so ill I'd be counting the hours until my next beta blocker dose, which seemed to calm the worst of the symptoms. I couldn't imagine how I'd ever be able to stop taking them.

At some point amidst all this I'd stumbled across the Long Haul Covid Fighters Facebook group and it had become my lifeline. If I'd thought I was the only person having these bizarre symptoms I might have had less confidence to try to ride them out each time and may have ended up in hospital. However, I now knew that thousands of other people were having similar symptoms and searching for ways to help themselves, as I was. Despite my determination to stay out of hospital, every few weeks a symptom would become so worrying that I'd have a sense that I'd crossed the thin line between managing my symptoms at home and becoming irresponsible. My bottom line was always that I needed to do whatever I could to stay around for the children as long as possible, which sometimes meant that I needed to get a particularly worrying symptom checked out. The increasing intensity of a particular symptom would take hold and force me to get myself to the last place I wanted to go – A&E. Each time I feared that I'd be whisked into hospital, swept up into the system, and I'd be unable to go home. Writing this, I feel foolish and naïve. I needn't have worried about that. I couldn't have been more wrong. Unknowingly I'd embarked on a parallel journey to that of Long Covid – the precarious journey of invisible illness.

NOTES

Chapter Two

Invisible Illness and the Healing Power of Being Believed

WHAT IS ILLNESS 'SUPPOSED' TO LOOK LIKE?

'You're looking well!' It must have been sometime between when I'd resurfaced from the worst of the waves of symptoms in the summer of 2020 and before my oxygen started dropping in the October. I'd made it out of the door and was aiming for a slow shuffle to the end of the road and back, my oximeter attached to my finger. I was embarrassed about how slowly I walked, so I'd avoid seeing anyone if I could. I also knew that if I got into conversation with anyone, standing still would result in my heart rate creeping up and up until I'd have to sit down to settle it, usually on the curb! Before getting ill, I hadn't realised how much of 'normal' life involves standing, but as my health slowly improved and I started to be able to go to the shop, I dreaded queues. I couldn't stand in them for any length of time, but I knew that if I tried to explain that to anyone I'd be unconvincing as I looked perfectly healthy.

I was shuffling slowly back home, not far from my garden when I passed a neighbour from the village. They'd probably heard on the grapevine that I'd been ill and wanted to acknowledge me in some way. I knew I'd have to pass them, so I engaged in a brief exchange of words while trying to keep my feet moving. I murmured something like 'thanks, yes, getting there...' and kept walking. I knew I looked 'well'. I'd put on two stone within a couple of months for no apparent reason.

It's still a mystery to me why I gained so much weight in such a short space of time. Of course, you'd expect to put on some weight when you go from exercising regularly to only moving between the bed and the sofa. However, it came on so quickly over a couple of months that I still believe that something else was going on in my body. Many people in the Long Covid Facebook groups are reporting significant weight fluctuations over short periods of time. At the time, the extra weight didn't really bother me. My appearance was pretty low on my priority list – getting through a day without some random alarming symptom was taking up a lot more space in my head than how I looked in my jeans and compression socks! How I felt about my weight did become more important to me as my health improved and I prioritised losing the weight. But when people told me I looked well, it jarred with the reality of how I felt inside my body. I knew I didn't look ill. It seemed I should have been looking thin, frail and vulnerable. Would people even believe me?

As Long Covid and its symptoms took hold, along with more trips to A&E, people believing my physical symptoms felt fundamental to my survival, both on a practical and emotional level. I needed medical professionals to believe me and take me seriously, especially as blood tests and ECGs were telling them that I was 'normal'. I also needed the support of my close relationships, as I could barely do anything for myself. I needed to be believed. I trawled the media for stories of people like me in an effort to feel visible. I was trapped in a cycle of times of hope, when a symptom would fade away and I'd believe that this time I really was getting better, inevitably followed by the increasingly familiar sense of dread as the breathlessness returned or my oxygen started dipping again. Being believed was fundamental to me getting out of this, and if I didn't look ill, or ill enough, where did that leave me?

THE TRAUMA OF INVISIBILITY AND NOT BEING BELIEVED

The sense of being invisible or not having my symptoms believed has at times felt almost as threatening as the illness itself. One of the biggest challenges facing many people with Long Covid and other chronic illnesses is getting people to take their symptoms seriously. This includes medical professionals and public figures in positions of power who influence public policy. In July 2021, a sociologist, Robert Dingwall, at that time a member of the government's Joint Committee on Vaccination and Immunisation (JCVI), claimed that any evidence for Long Covid is 'anecdotal' and that it may be that 'a lot of things are happening to a lot of people which are being connected in their minds with the virus but which may simply reflect the base rate in the population or some of the stressors that we've all been exposed to' (Newsnight 2021). People in positions of power are still making statements like this about Long Covid despite the increasing body of evidence of serious longer-term physical effects. Such statements undermine the legitimacy of people's illness experiences and create narratives which compromise people's attempts to access the help they need, whether it be medical, practical or financial. The extent to which illness is seen and believed has very real medical, practical, financial, physical, emotional and relational consequences. It affects every aspect of people's lives. If having the illness itself is tough, having to fight to have your symptoms believed is a further injury.

A sense of invisibility and sometimes a lack of belief in my symptoms has for me been part of the challenge of Long Covid since day one. More than two years on, there is still a failure to acknowledge the connection between so-called 'mild' illness and Long Covid despite there being clear evidence that many people with Long Covid were not hospitalised with the original infection. The narrative endures that Covid causes either severe illness which results in hospitalisation or death, or mild illness which barely touches you. At the time of writing, concern about a new variant, Omicron, is mounting and is being discussed in the media continually; not once have I heard Long Covid being mentioned as a concern.

My most distressing experiences of being disbelieved have been in face-to-face encounters with some medical professionals. As a white, female professional working for the NHS, I consider myself to be in a relatively privileged position. The odds of being taken seriously by other professionals are in my favour. However, several times I have found myself feeling powerless in front of a doctor who attributes my symptoms to physical manifestations of anxiety, and I've had little success with changing their minds. What chance would I have convincing them if I was anything other than a white professional?

The need to be seen and believed goes much further than the need to access medical or other practical help. Feeling invalidated or invisible can be intensely threatening to your identity and your sense of self. The extent to which we feel seen has a confirming or disconfirming effect on our own sense of legitimacy and authenticity. When our suffering is not seen or is invalidated by others, we learn not to speak it. Being silent cuts us off from the very thing which can help our healing – connection. Being silenced is lonely and isolating, particularly in the context of having a new illness without a path of diagnosis or treatment to follow from people who have gone before us.

THE GAP BETWEEN HOW YOU LOOK TO OTHERS AND THE REALITY OF THE SYMPTOMS

When it comes to talking with others about Long Covid, I've often felt as though I just don't know where to start, and often this keeps me from talking about it at all. It's like living on the inside of an experience which can't be seen from the outside or put into words – a sense that only people who've gone through it can 'know'. Work on illness narratives by Frank and Kaethe Weingarten has helped me to make sense of some of these feelings – why you might feel silenced if you have an illness which is poorly understood, not talked about or, in the case of Long Covid, new. Weingarten, in her paper, 'Making sense of illness narratives: Braiding theory, practice and the embodied life' (2001) describes how the 'cultural resonance' of a particular illness can influence the extent to which people in your life can engage with you about it in supportive ways (paragraph 'Narrative Closure'). The more familiar the illness, the higher the cultural resonance. Weingarten tells the story of her own daughter's rare genetic disorder, Beckwith Wiedemann Syndrome, with a low cultural resonance, 'Few people know how to respond when faced with the name of the disorder or even the names of the physical manifestations'. Having an illness with low cultural resonance can lead to a sense of isolation and not feeling understood.

Weingarten, in her discussion of Frank's (1995) classifications of illness narratives, describes how a 'restitution narrative' (paragraph 'Restitution, Chaos and Quest Narratives') of illness is perhaps the easiest for people to listen to and engage with:

> In the restitution illness narrative, the person tells about the details of the illness from the perspective of the diagnosis and treatment: all that has been done, is being done, and will be done if treatment fails. It is a story in which modern medicine is the subject and the star. (Weingarten 2001)

This story is most likely to be told about illnesses with which there is a known path to follow, through diagnosis and treatment. For people whose illnesses are not understood, such as those with HIV in the 80s, or people with ME/CFS, there are 'micro-processes of withdrawal' (Weingarten 2001) from medical personnel, family and friends to manage. If an illness can't be talked about in ways which are familiar to people, the person themselves may be marginalised.

Although, with Long Covid, the phrases 'long-hauler' or Long Covid were coined relatively early in the pandemic, what this actually means is still barely understood or often misunderstood, and the legitimacy of the condition is often openly doubted. It is easy to fall into silence where there is a feeling that no one can understand or that people may be sceptical about the legitimacy of your illness. In a pandemic where people are already physically distanced from each other this sense of isolation can intensify.

While Long Covid was just starting to be talked about in the media I was struggling to navigate the gap between how I looked on the outside and how my body felt on the inside. As well as my weight, I soon noticed other ways I didn't seem to fit the expected picture of an ill person. As I started lying on my front lawn instead of the sofa or bed, I gained some colour in my face and looked reasonably healthy from the outside. Close up I could see that I didn't look like myself, but not in ways that other people would necessarily notice. Over the months, as I started to make small, though unpredictable, improvements and I took tentative steps out into the world again, this seemed to only get more complicated. Even a year later, when I eventually started to appear out of the house, usually to pick up the children from school, I became increasingly conscious of the gap between how I felt and how I seemed to appear to other people. I felt that I was playing the role of a 'normally functioning' person. In some ways looking this way was an advantage as I drew less attention to myself. As far as others were concerned, I had disappeared to be ill for a few months and now I was back to normal – just like having a prolonged flu. At times I'd question my own perception of the illness. I would sometimes wonder if I was overreacting to the symptoms, as other people seemed to think I was better than I was. It was a bizarre sense of other people seeing a different version of me than the one I was experiencing, like looking in the mirror and having a completely different person looking back at you. Yet I knew I wasn't going mad; that it was real.

In the *Panorama* programme 'Long Covid: Will I ever get better?' (*Panorama* 2021), Lucy Adams (a BBC correspondent) and Susie (a nurse), had both had Long Covid for over a year at the time of filming, and discussed this in a tearful exchange. Susie talked about how she would push through the symptoms just to do basic tasks. People would see her and say things like 'you go out to the shops, don't you?' without seeing the disabling symptoms which would inevitably follow this one activity. Lucy also described how she would force herself to go for a bike ride to 'push through' but would be struggling to breathe during the ride and ended up in bed with a temperature. People seeing either of them would assume that they had recovered when in fact this one activity would lead to a relapse of symptoms.

This resonated highly for me as I felt that people saw episodes in which I resembled a 'normal' functioning person, yet this was just a façade. Every move or activity had to be budgeted for in terms of energy and resources. I was far from my normal self. My health, illness and abilities had become highly unreliable and unpredictable. If I overdid it, I'd 'pay' for it with a relapse of horrible symptoms. This created dilemmas which I wrote about in '100 days of Long Covid' (unpublished):

> If you have an illness which is unpredictable or can't be seen by others, you find yourself in a dilemma: if you push yourself to your limits to do basic tasks, or you're 'up and about', you give the impression that you're functioning almost normally. Relatively, you're achieving very little in terms of what you did before but now these basic tasks are pushing you to the limit. I was functioning at such a low level yet working harder than I'd ever worked. Sometimes it seemed pointless to keep fighting to do those small things. I was trying to stay positive and hopeful, but was there really any point? Working on staying upbeat and 'pushing through' wasn't working for me, and if I was to allow the darker thoughts to 'win' I could curl up in a corner, and perhaps be taken more seriously.

Looking back, I believe that those thoughts reflect the struggles I was facing with the chasm between how I looked to others and how I felt in my body. There was no one close to me who didn't believe I was ill, but it was hard for them to understand someone who could function in a particular way one day and then not the next. I didn't understand it myself; how could

I expect other people to? In Chapter 5, I explore further the possible effects on relationships of having an illness which isn't well understood by others.

THE HEALING POWER OF BEING BELIEVED

If feeling invisible, invalidated or disbelieved can push you into silence and isolation, in my view, being believed and validated can be a healing experience. I couldn't have predicted the power of having my symptoms taken seriously and legitimised, and the times that this has happened for me stand out as beacons of light during a very dark time.

The first time this happened was when I saw the GP I talked about in Chapter 1. She believed me and got beside me to help me decide what to do next. When I later reflected on that appointment in a conversation with her several weeks later, I wondered out loud how I got myself across the GP surgery and to her room. She responded, 'by sheer willpower'. I felt seen.

That first appointment was when I discovered the healing power of being believed and acknowledged. Until I really experienced my nervous system in crisis (which is now thought to be at least a part of the puzzle that is Long Covid) I hadn't truly felt the effects on my nervous system of being validated. This GP managed to tread the delicate line of talking with me as an equal, yet with knowledge and authority – exactly what I needed from a doctor at that point. Despite my vulnerable physical position, I didn't feel powerless, I felt safe. Rather than trying to 'know', which was, of course, impossible, she was open and clear about not having the answers but was willing to help me figure out how to manage my symptoms. I knew from the way she talked to me that she was starting from a position of believing me and it hadn't crossed her mind not to. I think this is what mattered most. It was a potent reminder of the degree of vulnerability you can feel when you are in the hands of a professional. The experience can be disconfirming or silencing, or it can spark connection. I didn't leave that appointment with a cure, or any real answers, but she did help me take a small but significant step towards healing.

One other experience with a medical professional stands out for me. After my first meeting with an A&E doctor which I described in the Introduction, I was extremely hesitant to return there when I had chest and heart pains which I couldn't ignore. Turning up to A&E became a regular occurrence over several months. A new symptom would appear and become increasingly worse until I felt I had no option but to get it checked out. Rather than risk meeting the same doctor again, I got my partner to drive me to a different hospital, further away, despite the fact that travelling in the car made me feel so much worse. I can still feel the creeping sense of dread driving up to hospital, knowing that it was the last place I wanted to be. This time the experience couldn't have been more different. I had the usual long wait and challenge of trying to stand in a queue to check in, which in reality meant me crouching on the floor in the queue, trying to avoid people's sideways glances! This time, the consultant was an older man who had an air of confidence but not arrogance – the kind of confidence that comes with experience and just puts you at ease. He did nothing different or special in terms of checking me out. I had the usual ECG and blood tests, from which, predictably with Long Covid, he found nothing concerning despite my frightening symptoms. However, he listened to me, talked with me and explained how little they knew about the longer-term effects of Covid. He explained that my ECG and other test results were reassuring, and that I should return to be checked over again if I needed to. He stayed to answer my questions and listened to my fears about my symptoms. I felt that he was really listening rather than trying to rush me out. These were all simple things, but if you're having serious symptoms such as heart and chest pains, being checked out, listened to, believed, acknowledged and told to come back if you need to, can be a powerful experience when you're in such a vulnerable position.

At that time, I didn't understand why my symptoms would start to ease after I'd had a positive experience of being taken seriously and my symptoms assessed. Now that I understand more about how Long Covid can affect the nervous system, it makes more sense.

When we are under stress, whether that stress comes from a physical or emotional source, our bodies respond by shifting into a 'fight-or-flight' state where the sympathetic nervous system is active. This prepares us to either fight danger or move away from it quickly by increasing heart and breathing rates and moving blood into the muscles and away from internal organs such as the liver and digestive system. In contrast, the parasympathetic, or 'rest and digest' branch of the nervous system, allows us to rest and recover from stress. It keeps us calm, lowers heart rate and allows us to breathe more slowly. At this time, I hadn't made the links between what I knew about the nervous system and what was happening to me. All I knew was that when I had my symptoms checked out by a medical professional who acknowledged my symptoms, something seemed to shift. I wasn't magically cured of all symptoms, but they did seem to calm. I had the sense of emerging from the other side of the latest tornado of symptoms.

This was not because the physical symptoms weren't 'real', but because the experiences of having my symptoms taken seriously and checked out helped me to shift from functioning predominantly in the sympathetic or 'fight-or-flight' mode of the nervous system to the parasympathetic mode. Twenty months later, I can often make a difference to my symptoms by deliberately taking steps to calm my nervous system.

My consultation with this doctor illustrates how the physical and emotional cannot be dealt with as though they are different systems, independent of each other. It was only with Long Covid that I experienced this on a primitive, bodily level.

Following each of these positive consultations with medical professionals, my partner commented how much better I seemed for a while after each experience. By this he meant physically better. Now that I understand more about the function of the nervous system, this makes more sense. I am not ruling out that other things were at play, such as the nature of symptoms with Long Covid, which often appear in 'waves'. It may be that these particular waves would have passed anyway by the time I'd been to the GP surgery, or come out the other side of A&E. There is still so much we don't know about Long Covid. However, I do know the difference these experiences made to my physical and emotional state. It wasn't that I felt a little better for having talked to someone, or that the person did anything that looked out of the ordinary. It was that these experiences felt as though they were healing in themselves.

There is a huge body of anecdotal evidence in Long Covid forums that balancing out these two sides of the nervous system helps people with their Long Covid symptoms, and this is being increasingly supported by scientific evidence pointing to a dysfunction of the autonomic nervous system in Long Covid (e.g., Dani *et al.* 2021). Chapter 8 explores some of the practical things you can do to help balance out the two branches of the nervous system.

I know that it is largely a matter of luck who you encounter when you look for help from a professional. The huge variability in the helpfulness of appointments when we consult professionals about Long Covid comes across clearly in online forums. In Chapter 7, I discuss how we might get the most from our consultations with professionals.

Although some of my consultations with medical professionals have been positive experiences, the more difficult ones made a different kind of difference. As weeks passed, it became clearer that no one really seemed to know how to help me. Most of my learning was coming from online communities of people all struggling with similar symptoms. Perhaps it shouldn't have been so surprising that as a community we were figuring things out for ourselves, since, as a collective, we were spending hundreds of thousands of hours searching for ways to ease symptoms, educating ourselves, reading studies and seeking out solutions. It started to dawn on me that the person who cared most about getting me better and who was going to do whatever was needed to get there wasn't a doctor, or any other professional. It wasn't even the people who loved me most in the world and wanted me to get better – it was, of course, me.

NOTES

Chapter Three

The Recovery Project

BECOMING YOUR OWN BEST ADVOCATE

The realisation that I was going to have to work out for myself what was happening in my body and what to do about it wasn't a sudden moment of clarity; rather a developing awareness that no one knew what was wrong with me and how to make it better. More than this, there wasn't the capacity to deal with people with these longer symptoms of Covid. In my previous life (before Covid), if I was ill, I'd go to the doctors with the confidence that they'd have at least some idea of what to do. But it wasn't just that they didn't know what to do. It was spring 2020 and the world was in the thick of the pandemic. There wasn't the capacity to deal with people whose lives didn't seem to be in immediate danger. Long Covid symptoms weren't even on the radar for a medical system trying to cope with a pandemic. The understanding at that time was that Covid lasted two weeks and if you survive that you get better, much like flu.

Long Covid is unpredictable and messy, much like the game of snakes and ladders that Professor Paul Garner compared it to in May 2020, in his article 'Covid-19 and fatigue – a game of snakes and ladders'. I'd like to tell you that the moment I realised that no one was going to sort this out for me I became my own hero, figured out what diet or magic supplements were going to turn things around, and got myself on the road to recovery. Of course, this didn't happen, but it wasn't for want of trying. Although there was never one 'lightbulb' moment when everything started to improve, there were small but significant things that happened which punctuated the endless fog of days, weeks and months. These moments are etched in my memory. Looking back, they were stand-out moments of clarity – beacons of light that each led to an unfolding of the next step.

The moment I realised that we were figuring it out for ourselves was one of these times. On one of those long, warm days in June 2020, I'd managed to get myself out onto the front lawn. Although I'd thought I was recovering, I was now getting waves of light-headedness when I stood up, and I wasn't functioning much at all. It felt as though it had been going on for weeks. Because I never had a cough or temperature, when I rang the Covid helpline about breathing difficulties I was told I had the wrong number and I didn't have Covid ('it only lasts two weeks'). I can see myself lying on the grass with the radio on, and hearing for the first time in mainstream media that some people were having some 'lingering' symptoms. This was the first moment of recognition of what was happening to me, and a disconcerting realisation – that we were ahead of the medical profession. When I say ahead, I mean that something serious was happening to my body that wasn't understood or even recognised by the medical profession. Many people in the Long Covid groups who did end up in hospital were being sent home to manage by themselves as often medical tests didn't show up any abnormalities. Although rumours of longer-lasting symptoms were starting to be discussed in the media, for many months discussions of longer-term effects were few and far between.

Realising I needed to do something to help myself wasn't some sort of heroic mission. If someone had been able to tell me what to do to improve my symptoms, I think I would have tried pretty much anything. Each time I found myself in A&E, I'd be told that my ECG or blood tests were 'normal'. As time went on, I had a growing sense of unease that each time nothing showed up on tests the legitimacy of my symptoms might start to be doubted. My biggest fear was that not only doctors, but the people closest to me would also start to doubt me. Becoming my own advocate came from desperation and lack of any other option. Yet it was also a fundamental turning point in my relationship with Long Covid. It was the point when I started to seek out things I could do to help myself. I couldn't let the thought that I might always be like this have any space in my mind. Staying like this wasn't an option – I had to find out what was happening to my body.

By becoming your own advocate, I absolutely don't mean dealing with everything by yourself, nor do I mean you can get better through effort, willpower or trying harder. Becoming my own advocate has only been possible through connection with others, and everything I've learned which has helped me has come from those connections. Each time I've learned something, it has led me to more ideas about what to do next, and to other people from whom I've learned something new. Long Covid isn't just an individual problem, it is also a societal and global problem. I hope that as research into Long Covid continues and we understand more about it, we will have increasing access to improved medical, financial and social support.

Becoming your own advocate is about you being in the best position to know what you need and want at any particular time and taking actions which help you get there. Being able to take some action has been fundamental for me in managing my Long Covid symptoms. That action may be tiny – perhaps something I know which helps ease a particular symptom or makes my day a little bit easier. Taking action makes a difference to how I feel physically and emotionally, and how hopeful I feel about the future.

One of the most useful things I have found to keep in mind is that *not a single person knows better than me how I feel in my body*. This helps me to make better decisions for my health every single day. If you take only one thing from this book, I hope it is this. We need the help of medical experts and people who want the best for us, but no one else, however well-intentioned, can know how you feel right now and what you might need. The stronger I get, the more demanding life becomes of me, and the more essential it becomes to hold onto this. That doesn't mean we always make the best decisions. If you're anything like me, you'll do too much and feel the consequences of that almost every day. Asking myself 'what do I need to do now/today?' has been and continues to be fundamentally important for me to make choices which support my healing.

THE IMPORTANCE OF SMALL ACTIONS

Being able to take some action in difficult circumstances can change your relationship with the problem – in this case, the illness. When we find ways of taking action, however small, we develop a sense of how to go forward and what next steps to take. In working with trauma, in narrative therapy there is the assumption that we always take some steps to respond to trauma, however small or insignificant these responses may seem. Michael White, the founder of narrative therapy, stated, 'Even in the face of overwhelming trauma, people take steps to try to protect and to preserve what they give value to' (White 2006, p.28). These steps, or responses, may be so small that they go unnoticed. They may seem insignificant, but by putting them into words and storying them, a person can start to discover or re-discover other versions of themselves. This can awaken a sense of agency, of being able to act on a situation, and lead to ideas about how to go forward and what next steps to take.

When I think about my earlier, most frightening days of Long Covid, it felt as though the symptoms were just happening to me; as though my body had been taken over by a sinister being. It was only through starting to gain as much knowledge as I could (one of my responses) that I started to feel like an active participant in my recovery. The more I found out, the less helpless and more hopeful I felt. Of course, that sense of fear every time a new symptom appeared didn't go away but finding I could respond in some way to the symptoms was a fundamental shift for me – there were things I could do to help myself. I started to glimpse previous versions of me that I recognised. Among them was the stubborn, determined me who could problem-solve and take one small practical step after another.

Over 18 months later, I also see that taking action was helping me to lower my stress levels and calm my nervous system. Being a restless, driven kind of person, I find resting, however important, can itself make me anxious and twitchy, as I want to be doing something more obvious to help myself. Being an active participant in my recovery by taking action became one way of managing the stress and frustration of being able to do so little and being unable to make myself better through sheer effort.

The importance of having a sense of control and being able to take action is well documented in health literature.

In 'Control beliefs: Health perspectives', Wallston (2001) explores the role of beliefs about control and how they can affect health behaviour and outcomes, where the greater the feeling of control, the more likely a person will behave in ways which lead to better outcomes.

MAKING RECOVERY YOUR PROJECT

At this point you might be agreeing in principle about the importance of being able to take action but wondering what to do in practice. It might be that you've already spent a long time looking for things which might help you. It was stumbling across one video made by Noah Greenspan at the Pulmonary Wellness Foundation (2020) that set me on the path to taking action. We'd gone to a stream where the boys could run around and I could still see them from the car or sit on the grass while they played. I'd stumbled upon the Pulmonary Wellness Foundation through a link on the Long Haul Covid Fighters Facebook group and I was watching one of Noah's Covid recovery videos. Noah was the first person I found who was really taking an interest in post-Covid symptoms. The video was describing the autonomic nervous system, and what can happen when it doesn't function as it should. In one slide, he described almost every symptom I was having. It's hard to put into words the excitement I felt; the feeling that, for the first time, someone 'got' it. Not only that, but he was helping people to do something about it. He was producing videos which helped people to understand what might be happening to their bodies, and he was developing a 'bootcamp' to work on regulating the nervous system. From then on, I was single-minded. Trying to recover became my job. For the first time there was someone whose guidance I could follow. Noah, of course, was completely oblivious to my existence and the difference he was making to me, but it didn't matter. His videos were giving me purpose and helping me to find each next step.

My days started to take on structure and routine. When I felt well enough, on the 'good' days, I'd watch his videos, read posts and articles from the Facebook group, and generally absorb everything I could get my hands on about the nervous system and breathing. I started to follow Noah's bootcamp. I couldn't always do the exercises as my symptoms would fluctuate day to day, but I adapted them to what I could manage at any particular time. At the same time, I was continually walking into dead-ends which got me nowhere. Someone would swear by a particular supplement and, desperate to believe that this might be the way out for me, I'd be online ordering whatever today's magic solution might be. Even if it seemed to make no discernible difference, once I'd started to take a new supplement, I was then too scared to stop it in case it was doing something important that I just wasn't aware of! But I was also developing routines and practices which became non-negotiable, prioritising these parts of my day over almost everything else, as these small practices seemed to be adding up to making a difference to my symptoms.

I believe that making recovery my project has not only had very real physical effects on my symptoms but has changed my relationship with Long Covid. Taking these actions gave me a sense of autonomy, of getting somewhere. It wasn't that I could always know what to do, or that it took away the fear that came with new symptoms, but it gave me the hope that I so desperately needed to get myself through each day, or sometimes each moment.

Prioritising and focusing solely on my health was a particular episode of this whole experience that has been Long

Covid. It was a moment in time when I was so ill that I could do little other than get through the day and try to figure out how to get better. I was fortunate enough to be on long-term sickness from my job as I could only do about 20 per cent of what I could do before. Although it was a particularly dark time in my life, I was to some degree, protected from many of the demands of 'real life'. I know that this is a privileged position compared to many people who have Long Covid, who have lost their jobs, or who don't have a partner to share the load. For a time, I was able to focus on trying to regain my health.

However, it soon became clear that there's only so long you can live alongside the 'real' world where everyone else is living. As my health improved, albeit unpredictably, erratically and at a snail's pace, I started to notice that the better I felt, the more the goalposts moved. Life expected more from me. It became clear that if I was going to stay on the path that I'd so carefully carved out for myself, I'd have to work out how to do so in the context of 'real' life.

FOR REFLECTION

- What one action could you take now/today/this evening to support your own healing?
- What might get in the way of doing this?
- What steps could you take to overcome these obstacles?

NOTES

Chapter Four

Recovery in the 'Real World'

For the majority of 2020, my world had shrunk to the walls of my bedroom, occasionally the lounge and, on a good day, the front lawn. Strange as it sounds, I'd almost forgotten I had a job. I often had to be reminded to send sick notes in. It was as though the 'me' that drove to work and spent 15 hours a day being busy with a real job and a real life was a completely different person. My job now was to get through the day, ride whatever symptoms came my way until my evening beta blocker dose, which seemed to calm my heart rate, and try to look as well as I could when the boys were around. Some days were quieter and calmer, and I was well enough to read or listen to podcasts. Days merged into weeks of functioning at a low base level punctuated by more severe symptoms and trips to A&E when things took more frightening turns.

Very gradually, the worst of the symptoms were fading. It happened as slowly as watching your children grow – you can't actually see it happening until you look back at photos from a year ago. The trips to A&E tailed off. I was functioning at a slightly better base rate. My routines of breathing exercises and very slow yoga stretches were shaping my days and weeks. I had developed a 'toolkit' of strategies to try to calm symptoms, and the symptoms had become familiar enough that I could often pre-empt them before they took hold. Something as seemingly small as hydrating before bed and as soon as I woke up (called 'front-loading') would help with the tremor I often felt in the mornings. After the drama of October 2020, when for a period of six weeks my oxygen levels kept dropping for no apparent reason, by January 2021 I seemed to have crossed an invisible line which I didn't even know was there. Without noticing, I seemed to have re-entered the world and its expectations. Although my body felt fragile and unpredictable on the inside, from the outside I looked better. The problem was that maintaining this basic level of functioning was taking every scrap of energy and willpower I had. What I was capable of from day to day was wildly unpredictable. I wasn't functioning well enough to proclaim myself better and participate in all that 'normal' life required of me. Nor was I ill in a consistent or visible way that was recognisable to others or validated by medicine. I was existing in a space somewhere between illness and wellness and I had no idea how to live in this new reality.

RESISTING 'URGENCY CULTURE'

Keeping myself at this new base level of functioning became my new job. It seemed to require me to somehow estimate what I thought I was capable of at any given time and to do only enough activity that I stopped before I reached the point of no return. If I did just slightly too much of anything, including talking, I'd end up back on the sofa, or in bed, often with palpitations, chestiness and a feeling as though someone had literally drained the energy from my body. One day I text my sister that I had a 'baffling cheeriness' (altered by predictive text from chestiness!). She replied, 'Baffling cheeriness?! Is that good?!' I didn't usually get any warning that I'd done too much and would often feel alright when I was actually doing something, only later to realise that I'd once again overdone it. I had very little capacity for anything other than trying to keep to my seemingly small but significant commitments to my health, which stretched me to my limits of functioning.

Living with chronic pain has been described as 'repeatedly switching between pain and other demands in the environment' (Eccleston & Crombez 1999, p.363, as cited in Weingarten 2013a, p.90). This description fits well with my experience of Long Covid. Living in a healthy body for me meant paying it little attention. It just did what I needed it to. With pain, disability or illness your body demands you to continually focus inwards – it demands your attention. Long Covid has meant a constant assessment and reassessment of external demands of the environment and how they fit with the internal needs of my body.

To the outside world I seemed better. There was no one particular person putting pressure on me to function, but I had a sense of unspoken expectation to be back to 'normal'. I kept reading about how important it is to rest, but there didn't seem to be much of a place in the world for resting. The Holistic Psychologist (2021) describes what she calls 'urgency culture', where productivity and busyness are highly valued and implied as measures of your worth. In practice, this might look like expectations to respond immediately to emails, texts or WhatsApp messages, and to be available or 'connected' at any time of the day (or night). These ideas about how things should be don't just exist out in the world, outside of us, but are often internalised, as though they are truths about how we should be functioning. As long as I can remember I've always been working towards a goal. I know how to do this, but I'm less good at slowing down or resting. Long Covid has forced me to slow down and sometimes stop, despite my continued resistance. The intrinsic value bound up with being busy has intensified with the demands of the fast-paced lives we live now, with 24-hour accessibility of many things, next-day delivery, and with online platforms which encourage us to display to the world an airbrushed snapshot of our perfect lives and our achievements. Whilst the world we live in cultivates these expectations, Long Covid and other chronic illnesses necessitate rest and careful managing of energy. This can be a cruel blow to people who have previously led active, productive lives in which our self-worth may be intrinsically bound up with what we can do and achieve. What happens when we are unable to participate in so many of the things that seem to be valued in our culture and bound up in how we value ourselves?

Making these expectations visible is an important step to being able to resist them, or at least to start to make choices about what we use our resources on and what we let go of. Noticing them isn't a one-off practice, as they are so bound up in Western culture. Perhaps cultivating a practice of asking ourselves questions, particularly when something seems to particularly jar with us, would be a place to start. We might ask: 'Is this a reasonable expectation of me at this time?' 'How important is it to me to do this?' 'How does it fit in with what matters most to me?'

We also play a part in setting up other peoples' expectations. If I send a text to my Mum, I don't expect her to reply quickly as I know she only switches on her phone every couple of days. Of course, there are particular contexts in which we have less choice, but there are many occasions where there is room for manoeuvre. This is easier when we are clearer with ourselves what we can and are willing to participate in and what we are not. Making these choices isn't always easy or comfortable, as they can mean stepping outside of norms and the expectations of others. Since I became more aware of my limits on the amount of incoming information I can manage, I have resisted joining certain WhatsApp groups. Making these choices sometimes sets me apart from other people and it's not always a comfortable place to be. However, I know that expectation to 'keep up' creates a stress on my nervous system which I've felt I can't afford if I'm to keep functioning as I am.

Weingarten uses the metaphor of the boatman's plight when working with people with chronic illness, joining them in working out what to keep in their boat or throw overboard each day (Weingarten 2013b). Imagine waking up each morning with a full boat and needing to decide what essential items to keep hold of and what to throw overboard. She explores the challenges of doing this, and how difficult it can be to decide which things of value to you can be thrown overboard that day. It requires an acknowledgement that we can't do everything we need or want to, or all that we did when we were well. I've found the boatman's plight metaphor a useful concept to keep in mind to balance the requirements of the day and the limitations of my own body.

PROGRESSION CULTURE

Bound up with urgency culture is the way in which progress is valued and held up as intrinsically admirable. From a very young age we are taught that being useful and reaching goals is to be valued, and we can internalise these as fundamental measures of our worth. Technology is providing us with more and more ways in which we can measure ourselves. Every Monday morning my phone tells me how well I've 'performed' over the last week. I get reports of my weekly step count and screen time, my fitness tracker tells me how much deep sleep I've managed and if I miss a day on my language app it sends me reminders not to ruin my 'streak'. If I ignore these reminders, I'm told that I've made it sad! Even my meditation app measures how many consecutive days I've managed to meditate. Of course, I am choosing to use these apps and devices, and like many people I've found devices such as a fitness tracker and a pulse oximeter incredibly helpful to track my health. However, I've found it to be a fine line as to whether I'm using the devices and apps to manage my health or whether they're managing me! At one point, I felt that the extent to which I was using my pulse oximeter was becoming unhelpful as I was checking it a lot and became quite anxious if I hadn't checked it, or if I had and the reading was low. I gradually found myself using it less as my health started to improve.

It can be so easy to get caught up in cultural ideas of what progress should look like. Resisting these ideas may require asking yourself, sometimes daily, or even several times a day, what is most important to you at any time, so that you can figure out what to send overboard. Pressures and expectations come not only from outside us, but from all the ideas and values which we take on throughout our lives, often without stopping to question how well they still fit for us. For me I have to keep reminding myself why it's so important for me to prioritise my health, and revisit these reasons over and over again, every time I'm tempted to do just one more thing.

PROGRESS – 'HOLDING IT LIGHTLY'

Since Long Covid, creating routines and practices which prioritise what's most important to me has been fundamental for me to feel that I have at least some say in my own life. These practices, outlined in Chapter 8, have also become important in helping me to keep symptoms at bay. However, despite my commitment to these practices, there were days and sometimes weeks when I just felt too tired, ill or fed up to keep up with them. Some days the very routines which would usually help me would cause me the most stress as I tried to keep up with them. The phrase 'holding it lightly' originates from meditation practice and kept coming into my mind when I was feeling trapped by my own routines. Although I was aiming to balance activity and rest within each day, perhaps balance could also be found across a broader timescale, within a week or a month. Sometimes just letting go for a bit seemed to be the best thing I could do for myself.

'Holding it lightly' could mean many different things. For me it meant giving myself a break rather than letting my own routines become a self-made trap. With Long Covid, my body sets the pace, not me. However hard it can be to live within these boundaries and restrictions, there seems to be little I can do about it. I know I need to create enough space and quiet to listen to what my body needs despite the pressures coming from other parts of my life. I often fail. It is difficult every day, but some days more than others. Remembering to hold my routines lightly has helped me to keep them in perspective and remember to keep in mind the bigger picture. Sometimes the most valuable thing I can do for myself today is to loosen my grip on the coping strategies that often serve me so well.

In this chapter I've explored how we might prioritise our health within the context of the culture in which we live. Illness doesn't happen to us in isolation, but within the context of the world we live in and the relationships in our lives. Prioritising health can be particularly challenging when symptoms aren't visible to other people, or we find ourselves living in the space between illness and wellness. The next chapter considers some of the challenges which illness, particularly within the context of a pandemic, can bring to our relationships.

FOR REFLECTION

- What do you need to throw overboard today to keep yourself afloat?
- What could you try to remember to 'hold lightly'?

NOTES

Chapter Five

Long Covid and Relationships

Illness and its effects play out within our relationships. When we face illness, we are threatened with the loss of the person we want to be. Illness narrows down our experiences, the things we can do, and opportunities for connecting with others. As our lives become thinned down, so do the ways we experience ourselves. We live the illness, talk about the illness, and people start to only ask us about the illness. It's no wonder that it can take over how we see ourselves and how other people experience us, or how we see ourselves through their eyes.

When I was able to do very little for my children, I started to look at myself through their eyes. I saw myself as lacking; not the mother I was wanting to be for them. If I couldn't even get up to make them a drink, how could I possibly be a good mother? I don't think this was important to them, they just wanted me there, but my experience of myself and my own mothering was one of inadequacy.

At the same time, Long Covid seemed to be causing trouble in other relationships. I felt alone in my experience, as though people just couldn't understand. I had a sense of being changed by what I'd gone through but couldn't find the words to describe it to anyone else. I barely understood it myself.

I frequently felt misunderstood or angry with other people's responses to Covid, which at times led to a sense of isolation.

As I was noticing the effects of Long Covid in my own life I was also reading about other people's struggles with the effects of Long Covid on their relationships. There were conversations about lost relationships, misunderstandings or people not seeming to understand just how ill Long Covid can make you. It sometimes felt to me as though only people who had Long Covid could understand.

This is not just about the 'big stuff' of relationships. It is often the small things that sneak into relationships and between people that become the 'big stuff'. A passing comment would make me think that someone who I thought understood was actually living in a different space and time to the one I was living in. Someone not seeming to understand how ill I was, or how hard I was working just to get through a day was indescribably painful. The seriousness of Long Covid being denied would ignite such an anger inside me. At times I was baffled by my own feelings. Why was it so difficult to find an answer to 'how are you?' Why did I feel as though I should say I'm getting better when I wasn't sure I was at all? Why was it so painful when people just didn't seem to understand?

While these questions aren't simple to answer, some of the work on narratives of illness from narrative therapy really helped me to make sense of these feelings and dilemmas. I'll explore some of these ideas in this chapter.

LONG COVID: AN INTENSELY PERSONAL GLOBAL EXPERIENCE

June 2021. A new strain of Covid is threatening the government's plans to 're-open' the country on June 21st. I once again find myself glued to *Newsnight*. Will social distancing rules be abolished so that the country can return to 'normal'? It seems that as long as the new strain is not leading to more hospitalisations and deaths then the country will 'open up'. I have to switch off. You'd think by now I'd have learned not to watch. Once again, Long Covid seems to be missing from the conversation. When it does come up in debates, it is often as an afterthought. Discussions on Long Covid might be more visible than a few months ago, but it seems conspicuously absent when making decisions around Covid. I can't help feeling that we're just collateral damage. But then to be viewed as collateral damage, surely you have to be seen in the first place?

It all felt so painfully personal. Whenever Long Covid was mentioned, I would instantly be on edge, like a raw nerve was being touched. I'd brace myself for whatever was to come and the feelings that would inevitably arise in me. They were talking about a global catastrophe, but it was as though the person talking about it was reaching into a most painful and personal part of me and my experience. Yet I seemed compelled to listen, whilst also preparing myself for the effect it would inevitably have on me. If Long Covid were ignored, I'd feel worse. A few times I found myself furiously typing out a message to a radio programme only for my message to go unread on air.

It's an odd thing when the cause of your illness is also affecting every other person in your own life as well as globally. No one escapes being affected in some way, often devastatingly so. Navigating day-to-day decisions about how to stay as safe as possible was a minefield through which everyone was having to make their own way. Important decisions about how to keep yourself and your family safe were being played out in the small day-to-day decisions. Everyone was constantly having to negotiate social relationships in ways we had never had to before, trying to work out what was right for us whilst taking into account other people's choices. It was like an awkward dance in which no one really knows the rules or consequences of particular decisions. Should my son go to the indoor party he's been invited to? Is it any riskier for him to go to the party than to school? Should we even be sending him to school? Everyone was having to navigate their relationships within this context. With Long Covid, the dread of re-infection, while still trying to recover from a previous infection months later, looms large. Covid was everywhere, yet it seemed no one was talking about Long Covid or what happens if you do have Long Covid and are re-infected. The clash of the personal and global while often feeling invisible is an unsettling and isolating place to live.

CLOSE RELATIONSHIPS: PARTNERS, FAMILY AND FRIENDS

When I read other people's stories of Long Covid causing trouble in their relationships, I noticed familiar themes around relationships with friends, family and partners which echoed some of my own experiences. When I was bed-bound, it was clear that I was ill. My symptoms were alarming and the priority for me and my partner was to get me through the day, and hopefully for me to eventually get better. At the time of the initial Covid infection we were drawn together in survival mode – we just had to look after the children. As the months passed, I was slowly able to do more, yet my abilities were constantly changing. I was continually having to make choices based on my capabilities at any particular time. I'd avoid activities which took too much out of me for the benefit they gave, as I wanted to 'save' my limited resources for the things I felt really mattered – usually putting the children to bed. As my health improved, it wasn't so much that I couldn't do something, but that doing that one thing could cost me so highly in terms of symptoms and energy. This continual calculation of cost–benefit is mostly invisible from the outside, but from inside the body it's exhausting and intensely frustrating. At times I just didn't want to hear myself say out loud yet again, that I couldn't do something, so I'd just avoid it. Looking back, I realise I was on a crash course in the complexities of pacing within the shifting sands of my capabilities at any given point, but most of this effort was invisible to anyone except me.

While I was learning this new and vital skill in getting through the day, my partner was having to pick up the slack of what I couldn't do. We were both working harder than we ever had. We were constantly having to negotiate our lives through the lens of my illness and through the small but also significant ways this played out in the day-to-day, ordinary things. We had misunderstandings and sometimes forgot that we were both working for the same thing. My own experiences seemed to be reflected in so many of the stories I was reading of people with Long Covid. It can be easy to forget when in the midst of illness that it is the illness that is the problem, not the individuals who are often working towards the same goal.

So many people with Long Covid have described how illness has shifted and re-shaped their relationships with friends and family. Some people have lost long-standing relationships while others face the challenges of maintaining relationships through the complexities of an illness which often doesn't seem to follow the rules of illness as we know it. The feeling that no one can understand my experience has led to miscommunications or avoidance on my part, as I've either been living in survival mode trying to manage symptoms, or unable to put into words where I've been. My sense that people just couldn't 'get it' further isolated me. Nobody saw how ill I was, so how could they possibly understand what had happened and how I was changed by those experiences?

Of course, no one can ever really know anyone else's experience. With Long Covid, there is the additional complexity of it being a new illness which isn't well understood. In addition to this, there was the physical separation caused by the pandemic. For a long time, we couldn't meet each other face-to-face. I couldn't physically manage the video calls that people were setting up, so my communications with the people with whom I'd normally navigate life were reduced to texts or emails. We were unable to witness each other's struggles close up, in person. This physical distance can allow space to get into relationships and misunderstandings to fill those gaps.

At the worst times I felt not known. The less I felt known, the less I would tell people and the more isolated I felt. It is only through re-connecting with the people who matter most to me that I have felt a renewed sense of knowing them and of being known myself. As it has become increasingly possible to meet in person, I've had some tearful conversations, and attempts to catch up on time lost. Many of my friends were living through all the challenges of a year in lockdown, which in some ways completely passed me by. These conversations have reminded me that not only do I have friends, but I can still be a friend – something which Long Covid seemed to separate me from. Through sharing stories, I've remembered who they are, and who I am beyond a person with Long Covid.

WHY 'HOW ARE YOU?' CAN BE SUCH A DIFFICULT QUESTION TO ANSWER

Sometimes the challenges that illness can bring into relationships can't be resolved so simply. I've read stories of people with Long Covid losing partners and friends or having these relationships seriously challenged because their illness isn't entirely believed. There may be ideas around that someone should be better within a particular timeframe, or that they could get better if they just tried harder. Facing these beliefs from others in our lives can be devastating.

When it comes to relationships within the context of illness, sometimes it has been the seemingly simple things that have baffled me the most. The simple question 'how are you?' could sometimes stun me into silence as I failed to find the words to form a reasonable response. Unless the query came from a close friend, I didn't think that anyone would want an honest answer. My usual response was something along the lines of 'oh, you know, getting there'. I seemed to say this a lot. Whenever I did, I had a strange sense of letting myself down, as though I was taking another step away from people and isolating myself further. I'd avoid responding to messages saying things like 'hope you're feeling better', or 'how are you now?', leaving them for when I might have the energy to work out what to say. I often couldn't give the answers that I thought people expected to hear – that I was getting better. I knew people were being kind and wanted to hear that I was improving. I felt guilty for wanting to avoid them, perhaps even a little embarrassed that I still hadn't managed to get better. Sometimes, saying 'oh, you know, getting there slowly...' felt okay enough. At least it was brief, and we could move on to a different topic of conversation.

Kaethe Weingarten's paper, 'Making sense of illness narratives: Braiding theory, practice and the embodied life' (2001) has helped me to make sense of why I was struggling to find the words to answer these questions. She explores how some stories of illness find an audience more easily than others, applying Gergen's descriptions of types of stories to illness (Gergen 1994, cited in Weingarten 2001). In Western cultures, a progressive illness narrative (Weingarten 2001, paragraph 'Stability, Progressive and Regressive Narratives'), where the theme is of improvement and recovery, is much easier to listen to than a regressive illness story, where things are getting worse. 'In my culture, the regressive narrative often produces isolation, both because the person who would tell it feels the potential of stigmatisation and marginalisation, as well as in the telling, the person is likely to experience both' (Weingarten 2001).

No wonder 'how are you?' was sometimes such a difficult question to answer! Most of the time I was avoiding thinking about the possibility of not getting better. Every time I was asked, and failed to tell a 'getting better', or progressive story, I also had to hear myself telling a regressive story and face up to the possibility of not recovering. Although these fears were ever-present, I wasn't always ready to entertain them consciously or try to put them into words.

The context of the pandemic adds a layer of complexity to sharing our stories of Long Covid. Whenever I talked about the effects of Long Covid, I was also talking about Covid – an ever-present threat in everyone's life. At times it seemed unfair to share my own experiences with anyone other than someone going through Long Covid themselves, and even then, there's always a risk that talking about aspects of my own experience will have a negative impact on someone else.

THE IMPORTANCE OF LANGUAGE

The narrative of individual improvement, as highlighted by Kaethe Weingarten (2001) that 'effort always pays off', is pervasive in Western culture. This narrative is wound into the language of illness – we are expected to 'fight' or 'battle' illness. It was as recently as October 2021 that graded exercise was removed from the recommendations for treating ME/CFS. Embedded in recommendations for graded exercise is the assumption that progressive effort will pay dividends. But with ME/CFS and Long Covid, exercise doesn't necessarily lead to improvement and can sometimes make things worse. So much of my effort goes into limiting activity. I'm constantly trying to pull myself back from the brink of doing too much – resisting going for a walk which might set me back or leaving that next load of washing which really needs doing but will push me too far. I always, always want to do more than my body is able, and I'm aware that a lot of this desire to 'do' comes from internalised ideas about striving to be fitter, healthier and better. Resisting exercise requires mental and emotional effort that is not visible to others and doesn't fit the brand of effort which is valued in our goal-driven culture. It's not glamorous and doesn't achieve fast or visible results but is fundamental in managing chronic illness.

The idea that effort pays off can be detrimental when played out in relationships, when people with chronic illness are being told that they have been ill for too long, that it's time to get better now, or that they would recover if they just tried harder. These narratives can be devastating; they can silence the person with the illness and distance them from the very support they need.

The language used about illness shapes how illness is played out in relationships. I've previously talked about how difficult I've found the word 'lingering' when used to describe Long Covid symptoms. To me, 'lingering' sounded like a few mildly troubling symptoms which may be difficult to shake off but likely to resolve themselves with a bit of patience. This didn't in any way fit with the constantly new, random and frightening symptoms which were causing havoc in my body. Language does not only reflect, but shapes how something is constructed in the world. 'Lingering' symptoms may be easier to dismiss, particularly when so many other people recover from Covid within a short space of time. Language can dismiss, invalidate and silence as much as it can be acknowledging and compassionate.

Perhaps one of the most difficult narratives to live through, and one of the most isolating, is the 'chaos' narrative (Frank 1995), named for obvious reasons. Weingarten (2001) describes part of her own experience of a chaos narrative after being diagnosed with breast cancer:

> this illness narrative feels like being in a kayak in a class five rapid. While you are going through the rapids, time and place shift so rapidly, up and down, right and left transpose so often, that one truly feels inside a vortex, the way out of which is entirely unknown in any one moment.

She describes how this narrative silenced her, through shame and rage. Chaos narratives are rarely seen in print, as it is only through shaping these stores with a non-chaotic mind that they can be formed into words. As Weingarten (2001) points out, 'what publisher would publish a book-length chaos illness narrative?'. Although I describe the overarching theme of my own Long Covid story as progressive, living through it in real time and from the inside has much more closely resembled a chaos narrative.

These illness narratives have helped me to make some sense of how illness can change the shape of our relationships and why talking about illness can feel so complex. These narratives aren't fixed: we are all the time moving in and out of them, often within the same illness, engaging with different narratives at different times. They have helped me to understand that I can share different stories of Long Covid with different audiences and still stay true to my own experience. Sometimes I need to do things which prioritise my health and people won't always understand, but I don't need to explain my actions to people. Perhaps I don't always need people to 'get it'. The narratives of illness have helped me to find a renewed compassion towards people who maybe did not know what to say to me, or how to ask, but were at least saying something. They have helped me to reflect on how I talk to other people about their experiences of illness – the illnesses which I know little or nothing about, and those that I'm tempted to think that I do.

This chapter has considered how illness can affect your relationships with other people. But how about your relationship with yourself? Illness not only gets in between people, but it can also disconnect you from the person you know yourself to be. The next chapter explores how the trauma of illness can affect our relationship with ourselves, and how we might begin to re-connect with the versions of us that illness may have distanced us from.

FOR REFLECTION

- How do you respond when someone asks you how you are when you don't feel like entering into a conversation?
- Are there any words or responses you could have ready for these times?

NOTES

Chapter Six

Responding to Trauma and Re-Connecting with What Matters to You

Between the 'waves' of symptoms I would sometimes make it to the car. We would drive out to a stream where the boys could run around and let off some steam. I remember my fear rising inside me the further we were from home, as I'd silently calculate how long it could take to get to a hospital if I needed to. I'm not sure when I stopped doing that.

The turmoil that Long Covid brings to your life isn't easy to translate into words, sentences and chapters. For months I felt numb to feelings. There didn't seem to be much time to feel. I was just surviving, holding my breath, getting through the day. Perhaps avoiding feeling was a necessary defence against something so overwhelming. Yet I wouldn't have described myself as traumatised; nor would I get a formal diagnosis of trauma. With time and distance, though, I can now see how traumatic those months were. Trauma isn't always loud, announcing itself abruptly, but can creep quietly, insidiously, under the radar. For so many people with Long Covid, in a pandemic which keeps us separate from each other, it has happened behind closed doors.

This chapter is about the trauma of Long Covid and how it can separate you, not only from other people, but from the versions of you that you know and recognise. It is not a chapter detailing descriptions of trauma, nor about re-living it – it is about how you might begin to re-connect with the you that Long Covid has tried to separate you from. It is also about hope. In the words of Kaethe Weingarten (2001):

> Illness is huge. Illness or, more accurately, our relationship to it, threatens the way we know ourselves and how others know us also. Anything that helps put illness in its place, which allows us to feel that we are who we are despite it, is welcome.

ANXIETY, DEPRESSION AND PSYCHOLOGISING ILLNESS

The intense feelings which Long Covid brought me, and which for so long I tried to avoid, could be described as fear, dread, anger and sadness. If you speak to a professional when you're ill, it's highly likely that you'll be asked about 'anxiety' and 'depression'. You might be asked to fill in a screening questionnaire for anxiety or depression. You may be unfortunate enough to be one of the many people with physical health problems to have your symptoms attributed solely to psychological causes. According to the Long Covid forums, this is happening over and over again, as it has for years for people with other illnesses where symptoms can't necessarily be seen. The word anxiety seems to have followed me about since that first visit to A&E. I'm asked about it, along with depression, in nearly every conversation I have with a professional about my symptoms of Long Covid. Yet for me, these words just don't fit.

As an observer, you might see the act of calculating how far you are from a hospital as a 'symptom' of anxiety. For me it was a rational response to a feeling that at any time something random and intensely frightening could happen to my body. At that time, I was ending up in A&E every few weeks with a new and frightening symptom. Yet all my medical tests would come back 'normal'.

Yes, at times I felt anxious, but really I was terrified. Dread, grief and despair were also frequent visitors at that time. I've never felt so frightened, wondering whether I'll make it through the night, or if I call an ambulance whether I'll ever get out of hospital. I've felt intense anger, with the government and media when Long Covid is barely mentioned in discussions about Covid and policymaking, with doctors who haven't believed my symptoms and with people who don't seem to take Covid seriously. I grieve what I used to be able to do and what I haven't got back. No one has asked me what it's like to have seemingly mystery symptoms which appear whenever they like, don't show up on medical tests and are often treated with scepticism, or what it's like living constantly with the threat all around you of the very thing that made you so ill in the first place. Illness exposes the illusion that we have control over our lives, and can lead to a sense of vulnerability that anything can happen to us at any point. Yet I just keep getting asked if I'm anxious.

The words anxiety and depression are descriptions, no more or less valuable than any other descriptions of feelings. But when I'm asked about anxiety or depression, I'm asked as though they are the source of the distress rather than an effect of living with an illness where you never know what's going to happen to your body next. This isn't just a problem of words and language – it affects how we are seen and what treatment or other help and support we can access. It puts the 'problem' within the person rather than being seen as rational, adaptive responses to a trauma, which make sense for survival. The anxiety I felt got me to the hospital that I desperately didn't want to go to. It helped me to seek out support and find ways to get through each symptom. Of course, anxiety can cause havoc if it takes too much of a hold on your life, but it is information to explore, rather than something to be treated as an illness separate from its context, as though feelings themselves are the problem. In her book, *Wintering*, Katherine May (2020, p.267) writes about how 'normal' feelings become monstrous when they're denied: 'There will be moments when we are riding high, and moments when we can't bear to get out of bed. Both are normal. Both, in fact, require a little perspective.' I may have been anxious at times, but it would have been odd if I hadn't. So many people with Long Covid and illnesses such as ME/CFS are being told that their symptoms are 'psychological', sometimes at the expense of serious physical symptoms being explored. Josie George, in her book, *A Still Life* (2021), captures this painfully and beautifully:

> I was asked again and again if I was depressed, anxious, but I wasn't particularly... My body was overreacting but my mind didn't seem to be... When new discharge letters came, they always mentioned if I'd cried. It wasn't illness or the lack of one that the doctors seemed to object to, it was the fact that I had feelings about it – as if feelings itself was the disorder. (location 2531–2542)

For me, a doctor appearing to view my physical symptoms as a psychological problem has felt like a nightmare where I'm shouting as loud as I can but I can't make myself heard. At one visit to A&E I felt viscerally the change in the room when my blood tests and ECG came back as 'normal'. The doctor went from concerned and curious to impatient and frustrated.

I had a sense that she had already left the room and moved onto the next patient. 'You've got two children...try and think of something else', she said, as though my symptoms were simply a way for me to pass the time, like I had a choice. Despite my inner protests, I often didn't feel well enough to even begin to try to challenge these statements, to change the mind of someone who'd already decided that there was nothing really wrong with me.

In Western medicine we have come to increasingly separate the mind and body into the physical and the psychological. Long Covid has shown me through bodily experience how our thoughts, emotions and physical experiences all work within the same system. Overextending myself in any way, whether physically, cognitively or emotionally, results in the same symptoms, and I can often calm them by getting back into my body and doing something physical to soothe my nervous system, such as breathing or yoga. The extent to which I can act on my own nervous system and calm my physical symptoms has been a revelation to me.

Long Covid hasn't given me a mental health condition which can be diagnosed and treated as though it is separate from what has happened to me, but it has taken me to some dark places. I have come to view what has happened to me as a trauma. The most overwhelming feelings for me have been fear and a sense of loss. When we go through something so fundamentally challenging as illness, particularly over a long period of time, these feelings can take up too much space in our lives, pushing out other versions of ourselves, the versions of ourselves we know or want to be. Our lives become smaller, narrower. We can lose touch with who we are beyond the person with the illness. Later on in this chapter I'll explore how we might re-connect with other parts of our identities which can get pushed aside by Long Covid.

First, I'm going to explore two of the most overwhelming themes which have run through my own story of Long Covid – fear and loss. If I were to try to draw themes from the conversations and stories I've read and participated in with other people with Long Covid, fear and loss would be the two which would come up again and again. How might we begin to make some sense of them and put them in their place so that we can make space for who we are beyond them?

HOW MIGHT WE RESPOND TO FEAR?

Long Covid is frightening – it has been since day one. I'm less frightened since my symptoms have improved and become more predictable and I have more resources to help myself. But the fear still occasionally takes me by surprise. If I do too much, what I call 'ghost' symptoms will crop up. They are like ghosts of past symptoms just passing through me, reminding me how terrifying they can be. With Covid still very much around, fear can also show up in situations where there are lots of people or when I feel particularly at risk. This morning, I was in a busy hospital waiting room for tests to check my lungs had recovered. I found myself continually weighing up how risky it might be to sit in a busy waiting room with people coming and going, versus the need to have the tests. The irony of risking possible reinfection to deal with the effects of Covid wasn't lost on me. While Covid is around, we are facing these dilemmas every day.

Fear is a rational response to a frightening situation and can help keep us safe. However, we also know that living in a state of fear over long periods of time isn't good for our nervous systems. Remaining curious about what fear might be saying to us can help us to find individual and collective responses to what frightens us. Since having Long Covid, I've found some simple ways to respond to fear which help keep it in check and from becoming overwhelming. I've realised just how much fear can grow in the dark, in isolation, when it isn't shared. We can take steps to manage fear on an individual basis but connecting with others has been the most effective way of diminishing fear for me. Below are four simple ways I have responded to fear in relation to Long Covid.

Getting symptoms checked out

This has been the single most effective way of calming my fears. For a long time, I didn't seek any medical help as I was so frightened of being taken into hospital at the peak of the pandemic. As soon as I'd talked about my symptoms I felt a huge sense of relief, a lot less afraid, and more able to respond to them. The times when doctors have taken my symptoms seriously have had significant healing effects on me, physically and emotionally. Even when things haven't gone so well in A&E, I've still gained reassurance from being checked out physically. I found that having a frightening symptom assessed by a professional can be incredibly effective in freeing you from the turmoil of going back and forth in your mind trying to decide how much you should worry about it. As much as I dreaded going to A&E, getting checked out calmed my nervous system and the next time I had that particular symptom I'd have the reassurance that it had been recently checked.

Doing your research

Similarly, researching and learning about my symptoms has helped me to respond to them and given me a sense of agency. It's wise to watch what you're taking in and the effect it's having on you, as it is all too easy to start reading frightening articles or stories which can have the opposite effect. However, it's also through research that I've stumbled across websites like the Pulmonary Wellness Foundation and Dysautonomia International, whose resources have been invaluable to me. They have also sparked further connections which have all helped me to put together my 'toolkit' for managing symptoms (see Chapter 8).

Building a toolkit

Having a set of resources for managing Long Covid and its symptoms can help to calm the nervous system and, in turn, calm the symptoms. This can create a positive feedback loop of reduced symptoms leading to positive psychological effects leading to reduced symptoms. Having a 'toolkit' has not only helped me to manage symptoms in a practical way but has given me a sense of control over the Long Covid, which in itself helps to balance the nervous system. The strategies in Chapter 8 can help you to form your own. A toolkit also incorporates practices which when done regularly can help to keep the nervous system in balance, which may have a knock-on effect on symptoms. Your toolkit will be highly individual, depending on your symptoms, but the feeling that you can take action undermines the grip that fear can have on you when you don't know what to do next.

Sharing your fear

Isolation creates the ideal conditions for fear to grow. Whenever I've felt most afraid of a particular symptom, I've initially tried to keep it to myself, not wanting to alarm my partner, and hoping it goes away. This is a really ineffective way of managing fear! Each time, the fear would keep growing until eventually it seemed to take over me and I ended up blurting it out anyway! As soon as it was 'out there' we could start to decide together what to do about it, and its power started to fade. Sometimes sharing it in a Long Covid online forum (in my case the Long Haul Covid Fighters Facebook group) felt like the most helpful thing to do. Fear starts to fall away when you share it with someone else.

'SELF-LOSS'

I recently had a sudden, visceral reminder of the person I was before Long Covid when a song came on the radio and stopped me in my tracks. It was a song from a particularly happy, carefree time in my life and an instant portal to the person I used to be. Hearing this song was a momentary meeting of the sadness of what I'd lost with the sense of 'me-ness' that it awakened. For those three minutes, I was not me with Long Covid, I was just me. Long Covid wasn't the whole of me. This episode left me wondering how I could get closer to that version of me at other times. Long Covid had diminished my sense of who I was, taken away the versions of myself that I liked most and left me as a shadow of my old self. The more days I spent living Long Covid, unable to do most of the things that made me 'me', the less 'me' I felt. Worst of all, I hadn't even noticed how much of myself had been chipped away. It was only in this momentary re-connection with 'me' that I realised how far I'd moved away from that person and that I really noticed what I'd lost. I needed to find those other versions of me.

'Self-loss' (Roos 2002, cited in Weingarten 2013a) is well documented in illness literature. In 'The "cruel radiance of what is": Helping couples live with chronic illness' (2013a), Weingarten quotes from Broyard's (1993) essays, *Intoxicated by My Illness:* 'since illness diminishes the self, how does one keep from "falling out of love" with oneself?' (p.25).

Before Long Covid, I was a runner, a friend, a professional and an active, busy person, amongst many other things. At my most ill, I was hardly any of these things. I was a mother, but for months even this felt fragile, as I was unable to do most things which I associated with being a mother. Illness can separate us from so many things which make us who we are. If this goes on for too long, we can start to take on the identity of an ill person as the illness pushes aside other versions of us. Being unable to respond to some of my boys' most simple requests at times felt unbearable, and I started to imagine myself through their eyes. I was not being the mother I wanted to be for them. I also grieved the loss of the carefree childhood I'd wanted for them – one in which they didn't have to wash their hands all the time or avoid getting too close to people.

Losses which may not appear significant to other people can have real effects on how you see yourself. Losing the ability to exercise is one such loss I share with so many people with Long Covid. It wasn't until I stopped being able to exercise that I realised just how fundamental to my identity it was. Not only did it help me to manage stress, it gave me confidence and a sense of achievement. The freedom of just taking off around the lanes for a run gave me such a sense of joy, of being alive. Going to the gym was just what I did, part of my routine, but much more fundamentally, it was who I was. I miss that energy high, that buzz which comes after exercise, as well as the freedom I had in my body and the knowledge that my body would just do whatever I needed it to.

Despite the losses I've described, I haven't spent a lot of time feeling sad. I think the fear hasn't left much space for sadness. Perhaps my sadness has also been obscured by anger, or simply the need to manage the symptoms. It has felt easier to feel angry than sad. Perhaps my wonder at still being alive has in part obscured the sadness. Yet I often still feel sharply the losses of particular versions of me, the 'me' that could be all of these different people, not just the me with Long Covid.

How can we respond to these losses when we can't do the very things which made up who we were – the versions of ourselves that we want to be? I have found some ideas from narrative therapy invaluable in helping me to remember and keep connected to who I am beyond Long Covid.

CONNECTING WITH OTHERS

The author and journalist Elizabeth Day recently wrote (2021) that 'connection is the opposite of alienation'. My darkest times with Long Covid have been when I've felt disconnected with those close to me, yet as I explored in Chapter 5, Long Covid has made it difficult to keep close those very connections which sustain me. I feel that I'm not entirely the same person as before, but I haven't yet made complete sense of this myself, let alone tried to put it into words to someone else.

Finding and becoming a witness

Having your pain witnessed in a compassionate way can be a powerful antidote to the suffering and pain of not feeling seen. In his book, *Retelling the Stories of Our Lives*, David Denborough (2014) discusses the importance of finding an acknowledging witness for our experiences, as well as being a witness to other people. An acknowledging witness is someone with whom you feel seen. In her book, *The Lady's Handbook*

for Her Mysterious Illness, Sarah Ramey (2020) writes power-
fully about the importance of having a witness:

> it has become clear to me that suffering cannot abate
> until it has been deeply seen and heard…when you sys-
> tematically disenfranchise and stop listening to the trau-
> matized, the victimized, the suffering, *that* is when people
> become embittered… Often one finds that this type of
> perpetual victim has not been compassionately witnessed
> by the people who matter the most. Instead they have often
> been systematically unwitnessed by the people who matter
> the most. Not enough people have pressed a forehead to
> theirs and said, *Holy, fucking shit.* (location 4598–4612)

It can be difficult to find an acknowledging witness, particularly with an illness which is not well understood by other
people. With Long Covid I've often felt most understood by
someone going through the same symptom, often one which
I have found difficult to put into words. David Denborough's
book, *Retelling the Stories of Our Lives* (2014), reminded me that
a witness doesn't have to be someone right there, in the flesh.
He describes how powerful what he calls imagined audiences
can be when we're trying to take action against a difficulty in
our lives (pp.59–66). An imagined audience could be anyone
who you know would be supportive of you, perhaps someone
from your past. Asking yourself questions from the point of
view of someone else who knows you well can help you to
access knowledge about yourself from which you might have
become distanced and can give you ideas about ways to move
forward. Denborough (2014) suggests thinking of one step,
however small, you might have taken in the last few months
to make things better or help yourself in some way, and asking
yourself questions such as 'Who in my past would be least

surprised by me taking this step?', 'What does this person know about me or has seen me do which told them that this was so important to me?', and 'What might this person say to encourage me to keep going with this?' (Questions adapted from Denborough 2014, p.64). These questions have you witnessing yourself from someone else's point of view, drawing on the knowledge of someone who knows you well, without them having to be there.

Being an acknowledging witness to other peoples' struggles can also make a powerful difference to how you view yourself. When I've responded to someone's post in the Long Covid group in a way which seems to have been of value to them, I have experienced myself as something other than just 'me with the Long Covid'. I become someone who can still do something helpful and of value to someone else – there is a sense of the struggle having some meaning. Being a witness to others can bring you closer to your preferred versions of yourself, those which Long Covid has pushed aside. The next section introduces some playful but powerful ways of getting closer to those versions of you from which the trauma of Long Covid may have distanced you.

Who's on your team?

From when I first discovered people online who were having similar symptoms to me, one connection led to another. Gradually more and more people were contributing to the knowledge and skills I was learning, which were all helping me to manage the effects of Long Covid. Many of these people had no idea of the difference they were making to me, and sometimes didn't even know me at all. I realised I had developed a virtual team of people around me, my own Long Covid recovery team! It reminded me of the 'Team of Life' work developed by David Denborough and his colleagues (2008, cited in Denborough 2014), although I have adapted it and applied it in a way which makes sense to my own experience with Long Covid.

The Team of Life is a metaphor, a way of thinking about our lives as a club or a team. It is a playful yet powerful exercise of re-connection, prompting us to consider which relationships sustain us most through our lives, or in this case it might be who sustains you through Long Covid. These people may or may not know you, and they may not even be alive. I have used this metaphor in both a practical and a metaphorical sense. As well as the closest, most meaningful relationships with family and friends, my 'team' includes doctors such as the GP who helped me through the worst weeks of my symptoms; Noah Greenspan, who posted all the videos which taught me so much about Long Covid; and my Dad, who, although he died several years ago, I know would be proud of how I've got through such a difficult time. My team also includes 'Yoga with Adriene', whose online classes make an almost daily difference to me, and all the people whose podcasts I've listened to or whose books I've read which have helped me to make some sense out of the chaos. Many of these people don't know me, but each of them contributes to my life in significant ways. This is your unique team. There are no limits on who and what you can include. Denborough encourages thinking widely and creatively, perhaps including pets or people who inspire you, who tell you something about how you want to be or how to go forward. Asking ourselves questions about who we want on our team and what is most important to us can help sustain us through difficult times.

David Denborough describes the Team of Life in detail in his book, *Retelling the Stories of Our Lives* (2014), and there's a template for this exercise in the Appendix at the end of the book. It is not an exercise in being positive, or in ignoring the adverse effects of Long Covid. It can serve a practical purpose in gathering together the resources which make the most difference to you, which can be invaluable when you can't think straight about what might help you. It is also harder to feel alone and isolated when you have knowledge about who and what sustains you and keeps you going, and when this knowledge is made so visible. Through it, I have realised that I don't always need people to be there in person for me to feel connected and supported. These team members represent and speak to different aspects of your identity, connecting you with parts of yourself which may have been obscured by Long Covid.

WHAT GETS YOU THROUGH?

Sometimes it is the smallest things which get you closer to your preferred versions of yourself. For me, music is an instant portal to a different 'me', yet I still sometimes forget its power. What gets you through might be the tiny things that Long Covid hasn't touched and which you can still enjoy. For me this would be reading, audiobooks, podcasts, films and, more recently, short walks. At my most ill, these things were tiny and often hard to find. Lying on my yoga mat to do the smallest of movements or lying next to my children while they went to sleep became important reminders of who I was when I couldn't do much at all. This isn't to deny what has been lost, but is about finding those small things that you can do which remind you of who you are. They might be small or ordinary, but significant in connecting you with preferred versions of yourself.

Documenting your responses to Long Covid

How we respond to trauma tells us a lot about what is most important to us. In Chapter 4 I described Michael White's (2006) concept that when we face something traumatic, we take steps to prevent, or at least modify, the effects, based on what matters to us. However, unless we make our responses visible in some way, they can go unnoticed or are forgotten. Putting them into words can help us to keep connected to what matters most to us. Thinking about how we respond to trauma isn't about being positive or ignoring the effects of trauma. It is about integrating all the different stories about our experiences so that we are not defined by one single story about ourselves.

One of the key concepts in narrative therapy is that you are not the problem; the problem is the problem. Long Covid isn't all of me; it is a problem on which I can take some action. For a long time, I felt as though I couldn't do anything about the symptoms, and that I just had to wait for them to pass. Sometimes this was the case, but even then, I was rarely just waiting. I'd often be working incredibly hard to get through to the other side of them. I'd be reminding myself that they have passed before, that they are temporary, saying anything to myself that would get me through. In time I also found things that I could do to calm my nervous system which helped ease the symptoms or stopped them taking hold. I was always taking action, even when it didn't look like it from the outside. I've never worked harder than when my symptoms were at their worst. Below is a list of some of the things I was doing when to the outside world I might have looked as though I was doing very little:

- When I was going through a particularly frightening symptom, I would take it minute by minute, drawing on any resources I could such as regulating my breathing and continually reminding myself that I'd got through it before.

- I reached out to others with Long Covid, reading Facebook posts and sometimes responding to peoples' posts.
- I gathered as much information and knowledge as I could, reading books, watching videos, contacting any medical experts who appeared to be taking Long Covid seriously and trying on different hypotheses about Long Covid and what might help.
- I looked for support wherever I could find it.
- I committed to learning about breathing and maintained a regular breathing programme.
- I committed to a yoga practice whenever my body would let me, even if this was just lying on my mat.
- I challenged anyone who dismissed my symptoms including medical professionals. I ended conversations with people who didn't take me seriously and I sought out people who did.
- I left the house whenever possible, even if just to sit outside in the daylight or go along to pick up my children from school. I tried to participate in my sons' lives in whatever ways possible.
- Every day I assessed and estimated what resources I had, prioritised what mattered most and what I could let go, often reviewing this several times a day.

Writing this list tells me a lot about what matters most to me and what I've been doing to stay connected to these things. With Long Covid I've had to see myself in ways I never have before, but I've also been surprised by what I can survive and tolerate, and it has made clear what I want to spend my precious time doing. This doesn't take away the losses, but it shows me that they are not the only story.

It is so easy to overlook your own responses when they're not put into words. Writing down your responses to Long Covid or talking through them with someone else can be a way of re-connecting with versions of yourself which Long Covid may have obscured. The questions at the end of this chapter, some of which are inspired by David Denborough's (2014) book, *Retelling the Stories of Our Lives*, Chapters 3 and 7, are intended to help you make visible and document some of your own responses.

'Re-grading' rituals and celebrations

When it was approaching a year since my first Covid symptom I started having the urge to mark it in some way. I didn't entirely understand why, but it felt important to me. It wasn't for anyone else to witness particularly, but to acknowledge to myself that despite all that had happened, I was still here, and I wanted a cake to celebrate! I noticed that other people in the Facebook group were doing similar and marking the day, perhaps to announce 'I'm still here' or maybe as an act of defiance against Covid. Being a year on from getting Covid and still having some symptoms was a mix of sadness, loss and grief, but also a kind of wonder and sense of triumph at surviving the biggest challenge of my life. It made me think of the 're-grading' rituals described by Denborough (2014, p.77) as antidotes to the 'de-grading' rituals that he describes which 'make us feel useless, unimportant, or worse'. The powerlessness and hopelessness I experienced when my symptoms were dismissed certainly felt de-grading. Celebrating with a ritual says something about having survived and taking a stand against Long Covid.

I started this chapter looking at Long Covid as a trauma and exploring the fear and loss which such a challenging illness can bring about. I then explored how we might make our responses visible and get closer to the versions of ourselves from which Long Covid may have separated us. I hope that some of the ideas in this chapter have got you thinking about your own responses to Long Covid, what you hold most precious and how you might begin to re-connect with other versions of yourself which Long Covid has obscured. The next chapters are more practical, focusing on getting the most out of consultations with professionals and helping you to build your own 'toolkit' made up of the things which help you most.

FOR REFLECTION

Your responses to Long Covid

On the following pages are some questions to help prompt further thinking about how you've responded to the challenges of Long Covid and what next steps you might want to take. As there are quite a lot of questions, you might want to work through them over days or weeks, but I would suggest going through them in order and reaching at least the end of question 6 before you break off. It might be helpful to talk through the questions with someone or write down your answers as this can add richness to the stories. Detail and richness are important because trauma can narrow our experiences of ourselves and the world.

1. What are the biggest challenges you have faced with Long Covid?

_____

_____

_____

_____

2. What names would you give to these challenges? (e.g., fear, sadness, anger, anxiety)

_____

_____

_____

_____

3. What does Long Covid have you thinking and believing about yourself?

_____

_____

_____

_____

4. How does it convince you of these things about you? What tricks does it play to have you believing them?

_____

_____

_____

_____

5. What effects do believing these things have on you?

6. In what (big or small) ways have you seen yourself standing up to Long Covid?

7. What do each of these responses say about what is important to you and what you want to keep close to?

8. Who in your life, past or present, would be least surprised by your responses? What do they know about you or have seen you do which told them that this was important to you? What do they know about you that Long Covid doesn't?

9. What might this person say to encourage you to keep going?

_____

_____

_____

_____

10. Which things are more or less important to you since having Long Covid?

_____

_____

_____

_____

11. What small things have made a difference to you? Perhaps things which connect you with the person you want to be.

_____

_____

_____

_____

12. What does living a good life mean to you now? What do you value more? What do you value less?

_____

_____

_____

_____

13. What skills have you learned from dealing with Long Covid, or what have you got better at?

_____

_____

_____

_____

14. What have you learned that you want to take forward with you in your life?

_____

_____

_____

_____

15. What has Long Covid shown you that you want more of in your life?

_____

_____

_____

_____

16. What don't you miss about what life was like before?

_____

_____

_____

_____

17. What would you like to leave behind?

_____

_____

_____

_____

18. What rituals would you like to do to mark where you are now? What is it that you would most like to mark or celebrate?

_____

_____

_____

_____

19. What next steps are important for you to take? (big or small)

_____

_____

_____

_____

20. Why is it important for you to take these steps? What does it say about what matters to you in life?

_____

_____

_____

_____

21. Who or what in your life supports you in taking these steps?

_____

_____

_____

_____

22. What obstacles do you think you might run into? When might you be most likely to encounter them?

_____

_____

_____

_____

23. What preparations can you make to overcome them?

_____

_____

_____

_____

24. What do you know about yourself that you've learned from past challenges which will help you now and in the future?

_____

_____

_____

_____

NOTES

Chapter Seven

Talking with Professionals

Making the Most of Your Consultations

Becoming ill in the first wave of a global pandemic is a strange and challenging position in which to find yourself. Before Covid, I hadn't thought much about our expectations of science and medicine, and the extent to which we rely on medical professionals to have the answers for us. It was on that day in early summer 2020 that it struck me that there were no answers to what was happening to me and all the other people around the world who were experiencing these frightening symptoms following a Covid infection. Before then, I'd lived in what I now view as a privileged position – that of not giving my body much thought but just expecting it to do whatever I required of it. I probably gave it less attention than my car! In the Western world we have come to rely on medicine to have answers for us when we become ill, assuming that it will be there for us if we need it. With Long Covid I had to face the reality that medicine didn't yet have the answers I needed. It was only slowly becoming apparent that there was even a problem. No one seemed to understand how ill I was, and it was a sobering place to be.

By this point, along with the growing online community of people struggling with similar symptoms, I had started piecing together some theories about what might be happening to me. When I eventually started consulting medical professionals about my symptoms, whether it be a GP on the phone or a doctor when I found myself in A&E with the latest strange symptom, I'd pose my theories to them, including what I'd found out about POTS (Postural Orthostatic Tachycardia Syndrome) and dysautonomia. I'm not a medical doctor and my theories were based purely on a sense of fit between the combination of my symptoms and the theories I was reading about. Doctors weren't yet able to confirm or dismiss my theories, but sometimes I felt that they thought I'd been doing too much googling. Eighteen months on and dysregulation of the nervous system and POTS are being recognised widely as being a significant part of the puzzle that is Long Covid, but there is still a long way to go in piecing it together.

MANAGING YOUR OWN HEALTHCARE

It wasn't until I was facing the symptoms of Long Covid that I realised that I needed to take my health into my own hands. Before this, if I had a health problem, I'd turn up to a GP appointment giving little thought to what I wanted from it. I'd relay the symptoms to the doctor and assume that they would take it from there. I handed the responsibility of my health over to them with barely a second thought. Since becoming a health professional myself, I have given more thought to what I need and want from an appointment, and with Long Covid, the realisation that I need to take an active role in my own healthcare has only become clearer.

In previous chapters I have explored the effects of con-sultations with medical professionals at which I have felt dismissed or invalidated, and those when I have felt seen and taken seriously. Of course, whom we meet when we seek help from professionals is largely a matter of luck. When we enter a conversation or relationship with a professional, the extent to which we can have influence or power within that encounter or relationship depends on many complex factors which are beyond the scope of this chapter. Even when I have assumed myself to be in a relatively privileged position as a health professional, it has not been easy to make myself heard or get the outcome I've been hoping for from the appointment. I've often felt the need to get my message across quickly before I lose the attention of the doctor. I developed a sense of urgency that this might be my only chance to be listened to and get some help. Getting yourself to your GP surgery or to A&E when you're feeling unwell can be challenging enough in itself. Additional challenges such as worries about the symptoms, fear of not being taken seriously or trepidation about attend-ing busy public places during a pandemic mean that the more we can prepare for the consultation, the less likely we are to be thrown by factors beyond our control and the better chance we have of communicating what we need to during the consultation. This is more likely to lead to a satisfactory outcome from the appointment.

SEVEN KEY PRINCIPLES

From my experiences both as a patient and a professional, I've drawn together seven key principles to keep in mind when having a consultation with a professional. It won't always be possible to follow all of them, but it may be helpful to have considered them and to have them at the back of your mind. At a time when services are stretched to their limits, preparation for a consultation can help both you and the person you're consulting to be clear about what you need.

The seven principles are:

1. Ask yourself what you most want to get out of the appointment.
2. Document your symptoms.
3. Do your research.
4. Prepare.
5. Take notes or ask someone else to.
6. Ask questions.
7. Consider when to look for someone else.

1. Ask yourself what you most want to get out of the appointment

If I can't prepare in any other way, this is the one thing I try to ask myself before I go in. It really helps me to focus me on what matters most to me and what outcome I'm looking for. Useful questions to ask yourself might be, 'What do I want to happen as a result of this appointment?', 'What outcome will be good enough?', 'What would I be dissatisfied with?' These questions can be particularly helpful if you're requesting a particular referral or a scan and need to be clear about why you're asking for it. Of course, it might turn out that your particular request isn't appropriate, but if you're not clear about what you're hoping for it's easier to lose track in the moment and find yourself feeling unhappy with the outcome later on.

2. Document your symptoms

Keeping a log of symptoms can be useful for being able to see how they are changing over time. A log can also come in useful in the appointment itself. My attempts at logging symptoms have been quite hit and miss – I've never managed to be very consistent. When I have kept a record, it has been valuable in showing me how my symptoms have improved when I didn't feel that they were changing. Sometimes I hadn't noticed that a symptom had even got better until I looked back at the notes I'd kept. Keeping a log has also been useful for reporting my symptoms to doctors as I'd sometimes forget even quite significant symptoms.

3. Do your research

We often can't choose which professionals we see, and often we don't even know in advance who they may be. Where there is any element of choice, it can be useful to try to find out the particular interests of professionals. In the GP surgery I attend there is some flexibility to see a particular GP even if that may involve a longer wait. Likewise, if you're having to pay for healthcare it goes without saying that it's worth doing your research and looking for those who are particularly recommended by others.

4. Prepare

Making brief notes before an appointment can help you to avoid forgetting important points, help to keep you on track and give you confidence during the consultation. You might write down the symptoms you want to bring up, preferably in order of priority in case you run out of time, as well as notes on how the symptoms are affecting you, what your main concerns are about them and what actions you'd like the professional to take.

Since having had consultations where I felt my symptoms were being dismissed or attributed to a solely psychological cause, I've put more thought into how to respond to these ideas when they come up. When I haven't been prepared, I've stumbled my way through these conversations, often coming out of them feeling powerless. I haven't yet come up with one way to respond to these ideas, but it can be worth thinking in advance about ways you might respond if they do come up. It could be something like, 'yes, it's very anxiety-provoking having these symptoms, but I don't believe that it's anxiety causing them. I would like you to...'. I'd welcome other ideas for responses!

5. Take notes or ask someone else to

Since the pandemic began, it hasn't often been possible to take another person along to appointments, but this can be helpful to keep in mind when it does become possible. Having another person to help you remember or to take notes can be invaluable as it can be difficult to remember everything important that is said, particularly when you're under strain physically or emotionally.

6. Ask questions

This applies both during an appointment and after. You always have a right to ask questions or ask for clarification. Most professionals will be happy to discuss your questions with you. If a request for a referral is turned down, you can ask why. You also have a right to ask for a second opinion if you feel you need it.

7. Consider when to look for someone else

From the first difficult experience in A&E I discussed in the Introduction, I have wondered when to stay engaged in a conversation when I feel as though my symptoms are being dismissed, and when I'd be better seeking out another professional. Even when a doctor hasn't necessarily agreed with me, I have sometimes still managed to get a satisfactory outcome from the consultation. A few months ago, I felt that I needed a neurology referral, but a GP I consulted didn't think it was necessary. In the end we agreed to disagree about how necessary it was, but he still made the referral. In that instance it felt important for me to persevere, as the GP was listening to me and taking into account my opinion. At other times when I've felt that I'm not getting anywhere or if I just haven't felt able to try to convince someone of the validity of my symptoms, I have looked for another professional. Over time I've realised that it is usually quite clear when someone is starting from a position of taking your symptoms seriously.

In this chapter I've summarised seven key principles to consider when you're consulting a professional. Although these principles are simple in theory, I know from my own experience that it can be really difficult to do all these things, particularly when you're feeling ill or under strain physically or emotionally. Even if you can keep some of them in mind, some of the time, you're likely to be in a better position to get the most out of an appointment.

The next chapter explores the practical strategies and habits that I've found to be the most helpful in managing my

Long Covid symptoms, with the hope that they will contribute to your own Long Covid 'toolkit'.

NOTES

Chapter Eight

A Long Covid 'Toolkit'

From the day that I saw Noah Greenspan describing symptoms of dysautonomia on the Pulmonary Wellness Foundation website, I started to make some sense of what might be happening in my body. As the weeks passed, I was trying out anything that might help me that I was learning from professionals like Noah and from people in the Long Haul Covid Fighters Facebook group. By default, I was creating a 'toolkit' of strategies and practices. These practices were helping me tackle the symptoms or 'waves' of symptoms when they cropped up, and practising them regularly also appeared to be helping to keep the symptoms at bay in the first place. I seemed to have developed my own self-managed rehabilitation programme.

Not only have these strategies and practices helped me physically, but they have also been fundamental in giving me a sense of agency in relation to Long Covid. It goes without saying that these practices are not substitutes for professional investigations and medical interventions. As you know, having a worrying symptom checked out by a professional has been a priority for me and the reassurance gained from this has lessened the grip of fear that can take hold when symptoms arise.

If you've lived with Long Covid for any length of time, you've probably already developed your own strategies which help you through, however small they may seem. If not, here is as good a place to start as any. At the beginning of the pandemic, people with Long Covid were only finding out what helped their symptoms through a lot of trial and error, but two years later and counting, we have the benefit of other people's experience. We know that Long Covid isn't defined by one single set of symptoms, and to date over 200 possible symptoms have already been identified. However, despite individual differences, clear commonalities and patterns of symptoms are emerging, and by the time this book is in your hands, there is likely to be a lot more knowledge out there about Long Covid, symptoms and treatments.

As different strategies and combinations of strategies are likely to be more or less useful depending on the individual, I have only discussed here the things that I've found personally helpful. Fortunately, to date they are also the practices which seem to come up most frequently in Long Covid forums. I encourage you to explore further the areas which are most relevant to you, personalising and developing your own 'toolkit' as you go along. What helps is likely to change over time as your symptoms and health change, although there are certain practices, particularly those that calm the nervous system, which are just as important to me today as they were when I first discovered them. This section will briefly lay out my key, go-to practices which have made the most significant differences to me. Each area or strategy is described relatively briefly, particularly those topics which are early on in their research, but where possible I provide references for further reading and research which you can follow up if it seems particularly relevant to you.

THE NERVOUS SYSTEM – THE KEY?

Before I had Long Covid, I didn't give my nervous system a second thought. Discovering first-hand what it's like when it doesn't function as it should and, most importantly, the influence I can have over it, was like opening a door to a world that I didn't previously know was there. I learned that emotional stress and physical over-exertion can result in the same symptoms, but I can also change how I feel physically and emotionally by getting back into my body and practising strategies which calm my nervous system. Only through learning about the nervous system have I managed to make these links and take back some sense of control. Now there isn't a day that passes when I'm not tuned in to how well, or not, it seems to be functioning. The ability to take for granted that my body will cope with whatever's thrown at it is a significant loss. However, discovering just how much influence I can have over how I feel is a revelation. If you don't read anything else in this section, learning about the nervous system is likely to make a significant difference to how you feel in your body and how you manage the symptoms of Long Covid. This section will give a brief explanation of the workings of the nervous system, followed by suggestions for key interventions which I have found to make the most difference. For more detail, I found Consultant Cardiologist, Dr Boon Lim's YouTube video of a conversation with his patient, Natalie, discussing Long Covid, really helpful and accessible (OneWelbeck 2021).

The autonomic nervous system controls all the automatic functions in our bodies, including breathing, heart rate, reflexes, the immune system and blood pressure. There are two branches of the autonomic nervous system – the sympathetic nervous system (SNS), otherwise known as the 'fight or flight' mode, and the parasympathetic nervous system (PNS), or 'rest and digest' mode. The SNS is generally a quick response system to physical or psychological stress. It helps us to fight or escape any danger by increasing heart and breathing rates, increasing blood flow to our muscles and away from the digestive system. In contrast the PNS helps us to rest and recover by lowering our heart rate and moving blood to internal organs. The rest and digest mode also helps to regulate the immune system.

Balancing the two sides of the nervous system is fundamental to good health. Our bodies need to be in balance. Spending too much of our time in fight or flight mode can result in inflammation and poor health. We can bring the body back into balance by activating the PNS and bringing down the fight or flight response.

So, what has this got to do with Long Covid? Watching Noah Greenspan's videos about the symptoms associated with dysregulation of the nervous system (or dysautonomia) was like putting all the pieces of a jigsaw together for me. When he described the symptoms of dysautonomia it was the first time I felt that someone understood what was happening in my body. I was struck by how many of my symptoms he was describing, from the palpitations and tachycardia (increased heart rate) when I stood up to intense thirst, breathing problems, dizziness, stomach symptoms and brain fog. Even when I wasn't feeling particularly emotionally stressed, I would jump out of my skin if someone so much as closed a door. In the Long Covid forums I was reading so many stories like my own. Dr Boon Lim (One Welbeck 2021) describes autonomic nervous system dysfunction as a partial or full explanation for the 50–60 per cent of patients with Long Covid symptoms such as dizziness on standing, palpitations and tachycardia, and the Royal College of Physicians (Dani *et al.* 2021) has since stated that Long Covid 'may be related to a virus- or immune-mediated disruption of the autonomic nervous system resulting in orthostatic intolerance syndromes'. Learning about the nervous system was the beginning of my path to learning how to keep it in balance and, in turn, to having some influence over my symptoms.

LONG COVID AND POSTURAL ORTHOSTATIC TACHYCARDIA SYNDROME (POTS)

I soon learned that a particular group of symptoms I was having, as were many people with Long Covid, could be described as POTS. This is a type of dysautonomia where symptoms occur on standing or being upright and can include light-headedness, palpitations, shakiness, exercise intolerance, extreme fatigue and blurry vision, as well as many others. At that time, I could barely stand for a few seconds before these symptoms kicked in. I never got a diagnosis of POTS as when I was having these symptoms the relationship between Long Covid and dysautonomia wasn't commonly recognised. Although beta blockers helped me for several months until I felt I could slowly wean myself off them, I do still have to self-manage a milder form of the symptoms if I over-exert myself. At the end of this chapter, I've outlined some of the strategies I've found most helpful for managing my POTS symptoms. Websites such as potsuk.org and dysautonomiainternational.org are also great sources of information for managing symptoms of POTS and dysautonomia.

THE VAGUS NERVE AND WHY IT MATTERS SO MUCH

The vagus nerve is a long complex nerve which connects the brain to the tissues and organs of the body and is central to PNS function. The term 'vagus' comes from the Latin for 'wandering', as the nerve 'wanders' right through the body from the brainstem to the abdomen and is responsible for most of the controls of the PNS. The vagus nerve regulates the control of the heart, lungs, muscles in the throat, airway, liver, stomach, spleen, gallbladder, pancreas, kidneys and intestines. When I look at some of my symptoms from the worst months of having Long Covid, it seems no coincidence that the symptoms which I found the strangest and hardest to explain – such as strange sensations when swallowing and in my chest, problems raising my voice, and breathing and heart rate issues – all relate to functions which are controlled by the vagus nerve.

ACTIVATING THE VAGUS NERVE

Breathing and the Mount Sinai Stasis breathwork programme

Increasing evidence suggests that many people with Long Covid are experiencing some dysfunction of the nervous system. This is backed up by an abundance of anecdotal data from people with Long Covid who are finding that calming the nervous system is having positive effects on their symptoms. Improving the function of your vagus nerve can have significant effects on how your body manages physical and emotional stress.

In his book, *Activate Your Vagus Nerve* (2019), Dr Habib

states that 'The first and most common cause of dysfunctional signalling in the vagus nerve is dysfunctional breathing' (p.65). It seems that these days everyone is talking about the right way to breathe. However, James Nestor's book, *Breath* (2021), is a fascinating, eye-opening read which explores how the way we breathe has fundamental effects on our functioning. Learning about breathing has been key to discovering just how much influence I can have on my own health – so much more than Long Covid would have me believe.

Many of us are breathing 'incorrectly'. When we are born, we breathe automatically using the diaphragm, a thin muscle which separates the abdomen from the chest and contracts and relaxes when we breathe in and out. As we grow, many of the ways in which we live lead us to develop dysfunctional breathing patterns which result in weakening of the muscles and nerves of the diaphragm. We learn to breathe from the chest rather than from lower down using the diaphragm. If we don't use the lower part of our lungs, we lose out on precious oxygen needed by our bodies for all its functions, including muscle use and removing waste products. Learning how to breathe properly from the diaphragm is one of the most simple and effective things you can do for your own physical and emotional health. It is the quickest and most effective way of tapping into the parasympathetic rest and digest mode of the nervous system.

The second most fundamental difference you can make to your breathing is re-learning to breathe through your nose. Your nose is designed specifically for breathing in a way that your mouth isn't, yet we develop the habit of breathing through our mouths. Nose breathing has so many benefits including helping to increase oxygen circulation in the body and even aids the correct formation of the teeth and mouth. I believe that following the free online Stasis breathwork programme from Mount Sinai Medical Center made an important contribution to improving my health. Their post-Covid recovery programme is divided into several different shorter programmes depending on where you are in your recovery, and they build on each other gradually. As my health has improved and I've had to balance different demands on my time and resources, I've found it more difficult to carve out the length of time needed for the later parts of the programme. However, I've learned a lot of exercises from which I can select one or two each day, even if it's just for a few minutes, and use them as I need to. Although that's not ideal, life can get in the way of good intentions, and I've decided that it's better do a bit of something than not at all.

Yoga

Yoga and its potential benefits for the nervous system could have its own chapter or book. Depending on where you are now and how severe your symptoms are, doing any sort of yoga might seem highly unlikely. It seemed totally out of reach to me when I could barely lift my arms or get out of bed. Before Covid I was never particularly flexible – my version of yoga was low-key, but I did enjoy short online classes from YouTube, particularly 'Yoga with Adriene', who I think is accessible, fun and effective and throws out all the cliches about yoga. When the worst waves of Long Covid seemed to be passing, I tried to get back to some low-to-the-ground slow classes, but I found that I could barely do the breaths or stretches at the beginning of the class. I only persevered because the act of rolling out my yoga mat connected me with a glimpse of the person I used to be. I felt a small sense of comfort from just lying on my mat, doing anything I could, however small, but just being a part of this online community.

Yoga calms the mind, improves strength and flexibility, and regulates breathing. It can help the body manage stress by learning to hold and breathe through positions of stress. Pilates has similar benefits, although I have only started doing Pilates more recently for strengthening purposes (see the 'exercise' section that follows). Yoga has effects on me which can't easily be described in words. It is the tool I've stuck with most consistently since having Long Covid. I do it for between 15 and 30 minutes on four or five days a week, usually in whatever I happen to be wearing. It is about getting back into the body, interrupting the process of moving from one thing to the next all day without taking notice of how I'm doing, both in my body and emotionally. With Long Covid, continuing to 'do' without stopping to ask yourself how you are and what you need to do can have a high cost. For me there is something incredibly grounding about the ritual of rolling out my mat and creating a 'zone' where I know I'm going to spend the next 20 minutes, whatever else I need to do afterwards. The ritual creates a unique space, protected from the demands of the outside world. As someone who is often living in my head, I find it hard to meditate in stillness, but following instructions from the teacher is like a moving meditation, the focus needed to concentrate shuts out other intrusive thoughts. The psychologist Csikszentmihalyi (2008, cited in Risen 2021) called this 'flow' – a state of being fully immersed in an activity. Getting back into your body is key to calming the nervous system. The practice of yoga and the space it creates encourages me to observe and listen to what my body is telling me, and helps me to know what I need to do next. The shaman Jo Bowlby, in her conversation with Fearne Cotton (2021) on her Happy Place podcast, described stillness as a 'portal, not a destination'. For me this describes poignantly the value of a practice such as yoga. The value isn't only in the destination but in the practice itself and what it connects you to.

This is not to say that on the mat my thoughts don't run away with me. I often remember things I've forgotten to do, or start thinking about something irrelevant, but the practice keeps bringing me back. After 20 minutes of yoga, I often feel that things are manageable in a way I didn't before. I see these effects as signs that my nervous system is in a better state of balance. I also seem to sleep better when I've done some yoga in the day. This may be due to using my muscles, even in small ways, and the effect of calming the nervous system.

Yoga with Adriene has free yoga videos on YouTube which range from seven minutes long to full 60-minute classes. Her philosophy is to 'Find what feels good'. This encourages listening to what is happening in your body and adapting the practice to how you feel at any particular time. I often miss out certain moves which feel too much for me or replace them with something which feels better in my body. You can search for a class to suit you using any key words, some of my favourites being 'yoga to slow your roll', 'yoga for a dull moment' and 'yoga for comfort and nourishment'. More quirky titles include 'yoga for when you feel dead inside' and 'yoga for zombies'!

Since the beginning of the pandemic, Suzy Bolt has also been running online yoga classes for Long Covid, following her own experience of Long Covid. Suzy has established a supportive and popular yoga community for people with Long Covid. I joined some of her classes early on and would have carried on had I not already established my own routine.

Whether or not you follow yoga specifically for people with Long Covid symptoms, yoga is an enormously effective way to calm the nervous system and tune in to what your body and mind need at any particular time. Developing this habit of awareness of your body's needs is a fundamental skill in keeping your nervous system in balance and managing Long Covid.

Meditation

Meditation has been shown to have significant benefits on vagus nerve functioning. However, unless you already practise meditation it can be easy to think that you can't do it 'right'. I have previously assumed that I can't meditate as when I try to sit still, my mind fills up with all the things I need to do. Meditation has falsely become synonymous with emptying the mind, when the practice is more about noticing thoughts and returning to the present each time your mind wanders.

A few months after having Covid was the first time I'd tried to meditate in any consistent way. I was ready to try anything which might have a calming effect on my nervous system. I created a habit of following a short daily learn-to-meditate course on the Breethe app (one of many meditation apps available), usually after lunch. I felt that I benefited significantly from deliberately creating a pause in the middle of each day to be quiet. When I was well enough to get out with my family in the car but not actually go for walks, I would sit in the car and do my meditation practice. Although falling asleep isn't the aim of meditation, I remember Noah Greenspan saying in one of his videos on the Pulmonary Wellness Foundation website that if you're doing a relaxation or meditation practice and your head starts to nod, that's a sign that your PNS is kicking in. Although I haven't managed to keep up my practice every day, I do return to it when I feel that I might benefit from it. The Breethe app has a wide range of mediations including coffee meditations, moving meditations and practices for sleep, as well as 'learn to meditate' courses. Now, simply the sound of the background music when I switch it on immediately has a calming effect on me. It is a paid app, but many free meditation practices are available on YouTube.

Rest

Getting effective rest isn't as easy as it sounds. If you're someone who is used to being busy you might have given little thought to the meaning of good-quality rest. Getting enough quality sleep is also vital for health and the nervous system. I know that sleep problems are common with Long Covid, but I'm not exploring sleep in any detail here as there is a lot of information readily available about maximising quality sleep and addressing sleep problems.

It was only through reading discussions in the Long Covid group that I started to think about different types of rest and why just sleeping, watching TV or scrolling on your phone may not be giving you the rest you need. Saundra Dalton-Smith (2017, cited in Beddington 2021) writes in detail about the different types of rest we need. These are physical (this can be passive or active rest), mental, sensory, creative, emotional, social and spiritual. These ideas struck a chord for me when I became aware of the exhaustion I would feel following a 'Zoom' call or writing for half an hour. Now I'm more aware that physical, mental and emotional effort all draw from the same 'budget', I realise that I can't afford to keep 'overdrawing' without also putting something back in. I'm still not particularly good at budgeting my resources, but just knowing this helps me to be more aware of what I'm asking of myself on any one day and what I might need to do to balance out my nervous system.

Quiet

Finding time for quiet or rest may seem like similar practices, but I do believe there is a difference. It can sometimes get to ten o'clock at night before I realise that I'm hearing quiet for the first time that day. We have become so accustomed to noise that often we don't even notice it until it goes quiet. One of the effects of dysautonomia can be an increase in the sensitivity of your senses. For a long time, I found too much noise and light overwhelming – I still do at times. Life is busy, noisy and full-on but I do try to carve out little oases of peace, whether that's a short walk or half an hour to read when my children are asleep, to hear what quiet sounds like!

Managing stress

In previous chapters I've explored some of the stressors of living in cultures which put so much value on productivity and progress. We can become so accustomed to expectations to 'keep up' that they become invisible pressures which we take on in our own lives. Add to this health, financial, work and social challenges of living in a pandemic and it's not surprising that so many of us feel stressed and exhausted. Although some stress is necessary to keep us safe and motivate us, chronic, long-term stress can have detrimental effects on our health. Before Covid I used to just keep going, giving barely a second thought to how I was managing to keep up. It was only when my symptoms were at their worst and I had to raise my voice that I appreciated the physical effect of stress on my body. My heart rate shot up as though I'd suddenly started sprinting and I felt ill. Never before had I experienced the effect of stress in a such an immediately physical way.

Of course, we can't avoid stress entirely – it is just a part of life. What we can do is try to be aware of the stressors we are facing at any particular time and find ways of putting back in what we take out. By this I mean aiming to rebalance the system with deliberate attempts to move into 'rest and digest' mode. I get quickly exhausted when my nervous system is out of balance, and I don't always notice when I'm running in sympathetic mode until I stop and realise how drained I feel. The ways we manage stress are individual. For me it is about creating points in my day where I give myself the chance to notice how I'm doing, whether that's through yoga, meditation or going for a quiet walk.

The more strategies and 'tools' you have in your toolbox, whether that's talking to a friend, therapy, writing, listening to music or doing something which takes you out of your own head for a while, the more options you have to try when you need them.

Connecting with the small stuff

With something as frightening and all-consuming as Long Covid, it is easy to lose connection with the small things of day-to-day life. Since being ill, the small joys which can happen in a day have taken on a new significance for me. I now notice things which I used to move too fast to see. Perhaps this is an effect of living through something so threatening to your life and health, but for me these small things seem so much more valuable than they used to. These small joys can provide welcome little islands of retreat from the bigger challenges of living with Long Covid. I try to litter them throughout my week. For me they include a really good cup of coffee, uninterrupted time listening to a podcast or getting outside for a short walk before picking up my children from school. They may not solve the bigger issues, but the small ordinary things can provide welcome relief and richness to your life, as well as re-connecting you with the things which matter most to you.

Cold water therapy

Cold exposure can help to train the nervous system to adapt to stress in a controlled way. Cold water therapy has become increasingly popular since Wim Hof (2020), nicknamed the 'Iceman', became known for his methods of cold exposure. Immersing yourself in cold water activates your sympathetic nervous system, causing you to lose control of your breath, your heart rate to increase and your body to go into survival mode. Although this sounds counterintuitive, it is believed that regular exposure to cold in this way activates the PNS and strengthens the vagus nerve as you learn to breathe through the cold. Research suggests that regular cold exposure improves healing and reduces inflammation in the body.

Although cold water swimming has gained popularity recently, the simplest way of starting is to add a blast of cold water to the end of your shower, breathing slowly through the cold water and gradually increasing the time you spend in it. The Stasis programme includes a simple plan for building up the time you spend in cold water each week. It goes without saying to take precautions and don't go out cold water swimming alone.

My own relationship with cold water exposure has been inconsistent. I'm a bit of a fair weather (or mid-summer) cold water swimmer. Despite my inconsistency I have been surprised by my ability to build it up over time. I tend to only do it on my better days when I'm feeling most stable, as it doesn't feel right to me to challenge my system too much on the days when I'm already struggling, and it isn't necessarily recommended to do it every day. Many people speak of its benefits. I can't say whether or not it has made a longer-term difference to me, but I do feel more awake and alert when I do it.

Exercise

With Long Covid being such a new illness, it is too early to make generalisations about the effects of exercise on people with Long Covid. However, similarities are being drawn between Long Covid and ME/CFS. The role of exercise in managing ME/CFS has long been debated and is a contentious issue. Graded exercise therapy has now been removed from guidance by the National Institute for Health and Care Excellence (NICE 2021) for managing ME/CFS, following concern that it may be harmful to some people with ME/CFS. New guidelines suggest that an individualised approach should be used for managing symptoms of ME/CFS, as it is such a complex condition for which blanket recommendations should not be made. This is also likely to be a wise position to take in relation to Long Covid.

With exercise having previously been a big part of my life, I find myself particularly vulnerable to wanting to ignore resistance from my body to exercise, and just 'push through'. In our culture we are surrounded by messages that exercise is the best thing you can do for your body; that it is always beneficial and the more, the better. Of course, our bodies are designed for movement, and we know that being too sedentary can negatively affect health. However, with certain illnesses, the relationship between exercise and the body is more complex and exercising more or harder may be harmful to some people. Exercise can teach the body to deal with controlled levels of stress and learn recovery. However, it is just that – a stress that needs to be taken into account within your overall energy expenditure budget.

Over the last 18 months I've made many attempts at my own graded exercise programme. Early on, exercise was far from my mind as I couldn't stand up. However, each time I felt a bit better I would start all over again, walking around my garden and slowly building up over weeks to a short walk. Often, I'd feel okay at the time I was doing it, but later in the day I'd be completely floored and unable to do anything else. I finally realised that if I stopped forcing myself to go for walks, I actually felt a lot better and had more energy for other things. I started to save going for a walk for when I really wanted to and then I'd budget it into my day. This won't necessarily be the same for you, but for me it has consistently felt as though my body needs to build up exercise tolerance over a very long period of time and it won't be rushed, however much I want to rush it! My body still seems to have the final say in what I'm capable of doing.

Twenty months later, I do go for short walks and I love them, although I try to not go on two consecutive days if possible. I also try to keep in mind that exercise isn't always the best thing I can do for my health, and I have to balance any activity I do with adequate recovery and rest.

Building strength

A recent consultation with a GP who specialises in exercise therapy reminded me of the importance of strengthening muscles. Months of hardly moving will have resulted in significant deconditioning and muscle loss, and Pilates is an effective way to strengthen the whole body including the core muscles. Several months ago, I started to do Lottie Murphy's short online Pilates classes, many of which are free on YouTube, which are slowly building up my strength. Becoming physically stronger has helped me to feel as though I can cope with more on an emotional level. With POTS, increasing leg and core strength is particularly important as it can help improve blood return to the heart and brain. If you're able to cycle, even for just a few minutes, it can help strengthen these leg and core muscles. Potsuk.org has some reconditioning exercises on its website, and the Levine protocol is a re-conditioning programme for people with POTS recommended by cardiologists which can be found online.

Like most aspects of Long Covid, 'progress' or progression of activity levels is not likely to be straightforward. Individual symptoms, physical capabilities and previous relationship with exercise are all likely to impact what we are capable of and when. It is easy to get caught up in pushing ourselves to be back to how we were before Long Covid, yet there is still a lot to learn about how Long Covid affects the body. I do try to listen to my body and how it responds to exertion, but it remains difficult, and the inability to exercise for any length of time feels like a significant loss for me. With Long Covid it is important to stay closely in tune with how you're feeling, not just during exercise but following it and later on in the day and week, noticing the impact of the exercise itself as well as its cumulative effects. I would recommend a very cautious approach to any exercise alongside medical advice which is relevant to you and your particular symptoms.

Sunlight

Sunlight and daylight exposure is closely linked with how we sleep, affecting our bodies' awake and sleep patterns. Our internal clock, or circadian rhythms, work on a 24-hour cycle and respond to light and dark. Exposure to natural light helps to regulate circadian rhythms in a way that artificial light doesn't. It is recommended to seek out natural light several times a day if possible, but particularly in the mornings. I do try to get outside at some point every day, and if possible, somewhere surrounded by trees and nature. The benefits of being in nature or by the sea are becoming more widely researched and understood. Psychologist Dr Audrey Tang (2021) suggests that being in nature can help us heal faster than being inside, surrounded by concrete or internal walls. Anecdotally I know I feel better when I've spent some time outside, in nature or where possible by the sea.

These are all practices which have been found to regulate the nervous system and strengthen the vagus nerve, and which I have found most beneficial, even if I'm not entirely consistent with practising them. Other methods for activating the vagus nerve include gargling, humming, activating the gag reflex, listening to music, and laughter and social connection. Dr Navaz Habib's book, *Activate Your Vagus Nerve* (2019), is an accessible read if you want to learn more.

MEASURING RECOVERY: HEART RATE VARIABILITY (HRV)

Discovering that there was a way of measuring how well balanced my nervous system is at any particular time and how well my body had recovered from previous activity was another one of those lightbulb moments for me. It is important to balance activity with recovery, particularly in the context of chronic illness. Rest is vital for the body to recover and adapt to activity, and our ability to recover from any activity is highly individual. In the right circumstances, recovery can be trainable, meaning that our bodies can learn to recover from activity more effectively.

Heart Rate Variability (HRV) is different to measuring heart rate. It is a measure of the time between pumps of the heart. It gives us important information about autonomic health and the cardiovascular system. The more active your vagus nerve, the more variability there will be between beats. HRV gives a strong indication of how well rested and in balance your nervous system is and can help you to judge the resources available to you on any given day.

Several devices can measure HRV, but they can be expensive. I use the free Wattson Blue app on my phone each morning to give me some idea of the extent to which my body is rested and has recovered from the previous days. The Wattson Blue app takes into account several aspects of recovery including some self-reported measures to give you a score for the day. A measure of recovery is made from information about sleep duration and quality, resting heart and respiratory rates and HRV. It also records patterns across days and weeks to give you more information about the wider context. If I have a low score for the day, I can't necessarily change what I do, but I'm armed with information on whether I'm pushing myself too hard and need to back off a bit or add in a bit more rest time. Slow breathing with a longer exhale than inhale (e.g., inhale four counts, exhale six counts) can help to activate the PNS and increase HRV.

MANAGING POTS

I wanted to include a section specifically about POTS as I know that so many people with Long Covid have POTS symptoms. POTS has also been one of the biggest challenges of Long Covid for me. A lot of the strategies for managing POTS symptoms involve activating the vagus nerve and calming the nervous system. However, there are a few more strategies recommended for managing POTS which I found useful. As always, they're not a replacement for medical assessment and intervention, as some of the symptoms could signify other medical problems. Further information on managing POTS symptoms can be found online at potsuk.org and Dysautonomia International's website.

Hydration

How well the body is hydrated can significantly impact symptoms of POTS. I believe that when I was well hydrated, my symptoms were noticeably better controlled. In his video discussing Long Covid recovery with his patient, Natalie, Dr Boon Lim (2021) describes how when you stand up, blood pressure falls and blood volume goes into your lower limbs, emptying the heart of blood. Nerves sense that blood pressure is falling, which activates an adrenaline response, boosting the heart rate and causing blood vessels to squeeze blood back upwards. He suggests that Long Covid can reset the set point for blood pressure control. Running on adrenaline all day through standing up can make the brain hypervigilant and can cause sleep problems. If you're dehydrated, or hot, your blood volume decreases even further, causing POTS symptoms to worsen.

Different studies vary in the amount of water they recommend drinking each day, but recommendations are usually between two and three litres. I often found that my symptoms were worse in the morning, and I'd frequently wake up feeling shaky. Drinking a glass of water before getting out of bed (called front-loading) helped me to manage these symptoms. Front-loading replaces the fluid lost overnight from breathing, sweating and not taking in liquid for an extended number of hours.

Electrolytes

Electrolyte balance is important to maintain fluid balance in the body. For a long time, I found that water alone seemed to pass right through me, and my thirst felt unquenchable. When I discovered that coconut water contained electrolytes I didn't look back. Although coconut water was an acquired taste it quenched my thirst like nothing else and drinking it became the first thing I'd do when I was feeling ill. Although there may have been a psychological element to it, I wouldn't leave the house without a bottle of coconut water, and I do believe it had a positive effect on how I felt physically. Some people recommend sports drinks or other electrolyte supplements, but coconut water worked for me.

Salt

In the POTS literature and in the Long Covid group there are many discussions around the use of salt with POTS, as it can increase blood volume and pressure. However, PoTS UK states that too much salt can be dangerous particularly if you have high blood pressure or kidney or heart disease, as well as in children. Therefore, increased salt should only be taken if recommended by your doctor. I did use more salt on my food for some time, but I never took in more salt in any consistent way as I wasn't comfortable doing this without seeking advice from a doctor.

Beta blockers

I was prescribed beta blockers when I'd been having tachycardia for several hours and nothing else seemed to calm it down. However, according to PoTS UK (2020), there are no approved medicines specifically for the treatment of POTS. They are not recommended for everyone as they can make symptoms worse, so any treatment must be carefully tailored to the individual. I feel that they got me through some of my worst symptoms, although the first ones I tried seemed to be making my breathing difficulties worse, and I had to change to a 'cardio-selective' one. For several months they helped to calm the worst of the symptoms, and I'm grateful to have had them to help me through. What I didn't realise was how dependent on them I would feel. At times I would count the hours until my next dose as I could feel the effects wearing off. I couldn't imagine how I'd ever be able to come off them. However, a few months later when my heart symptoms had calmed down a lot, I was told by my GP and cardiologist that I could slowly wean off them (it can be dangerous to suddenly stop them). Even though the cardiologist suggested cutting down slowly over a couple of weeks, it actually took me three months. I'd cut a bit more off the tablet each week, as I was so worried about the effects stopping them might have on my body. Eventually I stopped taking them completely. I know that people have had varied experiences with them, some more successful than others. If I were in the same position again, I would still take them as I know how much they helped me, but I would do it with some caution, knowing how long it took me to come off them.

Compression

For over a year, compression socks became an unattractive but staple part of my daily wardrobe! Compression socks, tights, leggings or even abdominal binders can increase blood return to the heart and help with POTS symptoms. According to PoTS UK (2021), there isn't any research to prove that they can improve symptoms of POTS, but many people do report finding them helpful and I do feel that they helped me. You can find a variety of different types and colours online, and at least 30 mmHg compression is recommended. It is recommended that they're not worn at night.

Other strategies recommended for POTS

Other recommended strategies for managing POTS symptoms include eating regular meals, keeping cool where possible, avoiding alcohol and sleeping with the head of the bed elevated, as well as making sure you move slowly when you go from seated to standing.

Things which would set off my POTS symptoms would be hot baths or showers (POTS symptoms often get worse in hot environments) or having to stand for any length of time. I found that my symptoms were worse if I didn't eat regularly, and for a long time I couldn't tolerate any alcohol at all, which fortunately has changed a little!

OTHER AREAS FOR RESEARCH

In this chapter I've wanted to draw together the practical things which have helped me the most with my symptoms, rather than trying to mention everything that is covered in Long Covid groups or other literature. The following are a couple of areas that I haven't included in the sections on the nervous system and POTS, but which I've experimented with, and may be of interest to you to follow up further, especially as research develops in these areas.

Food and diet

Although dysfunction in the nervous system is likely to be a major part of the puzzle of Long Covid, research is all the time developing theories about the causes of Long Covid and why symptoms persist. Theories include hyper-inflammation mediated by Mast Cell Activation Syndrome (MCAS) (Weinstock *et al.* 2021). Many discussions about food and what types of diet might help ease symptoms can be found in Long Covid forums. Personally, I haven't followed any particular diet or cut out any food groups. This has mainly been because I felt overwhelmed by different ideas about what might be helpful. I also felt that I had so much to think about already that restricting my diet in any significant way just didn't fit for me. I've tried to follow a generally healthy diet of fresh food where possible. However, many people in the Long Covid forums have reported following particular diets and finding that they help their symptoms. Dr Tina Peers discusses Long Covid, MCAS and histamine intolerance on a video with RUN-DMC/ Gez Medinger on YouTube (2020), where she talks about food, diet and supplements.

Supplements

Whether or not to take supplements and if so, which to take, is a subject which I've found difficult to navigate through Long Covid. I've read about so people's experiences with various supplements and many a time I've been tempted by a post suggesting that a particular supplement has had an amazing effect on someone's symptoms, and found myself buying an expensive supplement, 'just in case' it works. Over time and after a lot of research, I've settled on a few, including a general multivitamin as well as B vitamins and turmeric, but I think what you take has to be an individual decision based on thorough research. I've found that once I start taking a supplement, I find it very difficult to stop as even if I'm not clear about ways in which I'm benefiting from it, I'm also wary of stopping taking it! This has made me cautious and careful to do a lot of research before adding a regular supplement to my diet as the list only seems to get longer!

Hormones

While I'm not in a position to explore in any detail the role of hormones in Long Covid, research on the relationship between hormones and Long Covid is all the time unfolding. For some time, anecdotal evidence from Long Covid groups has suggested a relationship between Long Covid and hormones. Dr Newson's study on the role of hormones in Long Covid found that the mean age of people with Long Covid is 46.5 years, with 82.8 per cent being females. In this study, 36 per cent of women reported disturbances to their menstrual cycles (Newson, Lewis & O'Hara, 2021). Stewart and colleagues (2021) propose an asymmetry in risk and outcomes of Long Covid between sexes, an overlap of symptoms of Long Covid with perimenopause and menopause, and suggest sex hormone differences be further investigated. As many women report, I've noticed that my Long Covid symptoms seem to be worse at particular points in my cycle. While it is still early days for research on Long Covid and hormones, Suzy Bolt explores the subject in her YouTube video with doctors Tanya Patrick and Claire Phipps (Yoga for Long Covid with Suzy Bolt 360mindbodysoul 2021). Unfortunately, specialists in this area are often in private healthcare. If you notice links between your symptoms and menstrual cycle it might be worth tracking symptoms and hormonal cycles. I've found Newson's free app, Balance, helpful for doing this.

In this chapter I've summarised the things I've found most helpful in managing Long Covid symptoms as well as the practices that help to keep my nervous system balanced. These practices and routines form my 'Long Covid toolkit'. Some things such as yoga, I do most days, whereas other 'tools' I just use when I need to. Some of them including compression socks, beta blockers and coconut water I no longer use, but at a particular time they were significant in managing my symptoms. You may already be using certain tools, but I hope at least some of these things will be helpful for you to add to your own Long Covid toolkit, or at least be worth further exploration.

The next chapter discusses pacing – a fundamental practice in managing Long Covid symptoms. Because pacing can be so important in managing Long Covid symptoms, yet be so difficult to do in practice, the next chapter explores in detail what I see as the elusive art of pacing!

FOR REFLECTION

- What small things bring richness to your daily life or connect you with the person you want to be? Are there any that you'd like to prioritise including more of in your days?
- Which tools or practices from this chapter resonate with you most and would you most like to explore further?
- What next steps are you going to take to do this?

NOTES

Chapter Nine

Pacing

Before Long Covid, rushing around without giving a second thought to how my body would cope was a privilege I didn't know I had. As long as I can remember I've been someone who goes from one activity to the next, struggles to sit down or relax until 'everything' is done (it never is), has to do something straight away if it has entered my head, and who thrives when setting goals and getting things done. The enforced slowing down and, for a long time, being almost completely unable to function in a way that I recognised, was one of the hardest challenges of Long Covid for me. It still is at times. In previous chapters I've explored the enormity of the loss of the capacity to take for granted that your body will do what you want it to. I know that so many people with Long Covid are facing this. Many people in the forums have talked of being a previously very active, high-achieving person. Before Long Covid, pacing was something that I knew a little about through my work, but I had no idea just how hard it can be in practice. It is a way of proactively managing your activity levels so that you don't over-exert yourself, and is an important strategy for managing long-term health conditions such as ME/CFS. It didn't sound like something I wanted to have to do or see myself having to do over any length of time. However, with Long Covid all you need to do is ignore pacing for a day to find out how important it is. Pacing seems to be a lesson that with Long Covid, unless we take notice, we are forced to face, over and over again.

Literature from years of research in chronic illness, particularly in ME/CFS, has provided a wealth of knowledge and resources about pacing which are now informing resources on managing Long Covid. Longcovid.physio has a lot of information and links you can follow to learn more about pacing, and a simple search online can locate many different strategies for pacing. I'm not going to cover these in this chapter as they are so readily available elsewhere. This chapter is about the small things – the tricks that I stumbled upon and wished I'd discovered earlier. They're unlikely to be new, but they are small things which I haven't necessarily read about but have just picked up through trial and error, usually from doing too much and having to pick myself up once again. What works best for you is likely to be highly individual, but I hope you get something from me sharing what has worked for me. I'd welcome any other tips or contributions to add to these!

The aim of pacing is to avoid the 'boom and bust' cycle, whereby on a 'good' day you experience more energy and feel capable of doing more, so you do too much, drain your energy and resources, and often experience increased symptoms. You then have to spend a lot longer getting back to your baseline, or how you were before you overdid it. I have done this over and over again, as the temptation to go for it on a good day can be just too hard to resist. I know I'm not alone in this. Pacing is a daily challenge in which the goalposts constantly move. To me it feels almost like an art, finding balance over the day and week when symptoms may be changing all the time. I think very few days pass when I don't feel that I've overdone it in some way.

Noah Greenspan (2020) on the Pulmonary Wellness Foundation website gave one of the most helpful explanations of pacing I've come across. He describes how, with Long Covid, you have a 'budget' for what you can do. This accounts for physical, mental and emotional expenditure. The key point is that *all of these come from the same budget.* If you 'spend' 50 per cent on physical tasks, and then spend another 30 per cent on mental or cognitive tasks like reading, concentrating and thinking, and then you have an argument with your partner or have to tell your children off, you can tip over into overspending. Even 'positive' emotions like excitement draw from your budget. Physical, cognitive and emotional activity or effort all affect the nervous system and overspending can trigger symptoms. When my symptoms were at their worst, becoming upset or angry could trigger heart symptoms. My experiences were echoed in the Long Covid group. Some people would say that getting angry or upset would lead to a relapse of symptoms. It makes sense that anything which affects the balance of the sympathetic and parasympathetic nervous system will likely have an effect on symptoms, no matter whether the trigger is physical, cognitive or emotional. Pacing helps to keep the nervous system in balance. Below are the small but often significant things which have made the most difference to me in trying to pace my energy and resources.

RECOGNISING 'ACTIVITY'

You can't pace yourself if you're not aware of the activities that are taking from your energy budget. This relates particularly to the small things which you may not necessarily notice but can add up to a lot of activity. For me, being in the house all day falls into this category. Even if I'm not doing anything that looks particularly demanding, just being in the house can have a drip, drip effect on my energy level, yet I don't realise it until much later in the day. When I'm in the house I'm doing a lot of bending down, picking things up, doing one small thing followed by another small thing, punctuated by multi-tasking different requests from my children and forgetting to actually take any real rest at all. Going out might register more steps on my fitness tracker but leave me less exhausted in total once I've spent a couple of hours sitting in the car (as a passenger – for me, driving takes a lot out of the budget). Your 'drip drip' activities may be different to mine, but it is important to recognise them when trying to pace yourself, as well as recognising how much activities such as thinking, concentrating, using screens and talking can draw from your budget. Without that awareness it's so much easier to fall into the same traps each day.

THE DANGER OF 'JUST'

One of the most challenging aspects of pacing for me is stopping activity once I've started. I intend to do one thing, but then I 'just' see that other thing which needs doing and won't take long, but I'll 'just' stick a wash on before I sit down. Before I know it, I'm starting to get those horrible feelings which hint that I might have done a bit too much. These feelings later become symptoms, by which time I'll have to stop doing anything at all. I might not even be able to function at my baseline level for the next few days.

I now try to avoid running activities together if at all possible. It doesn't sound like rocket science but it's *so hard to do!* Temptations to just do the next small thing are everywhere. As long as I need to pace myself, I think this will always be a challenge, but I tell myself that being aware of it is being halfway there.

SETTING A TIMER

I've found setting a timer useful for managing the 'justs'. I used it quite a lot at one point, but I often forget now how useful it can be. It isn't an exact science, as what you're capable of doing at any point will vary depending on a multitude of factors, including how you're feeling on the day, what you did yesterday, hormones, hydration and what the task involves. However, setting a timer can help to remind you to stop an activity and take a rest even if you haven't finished what you're doing, otherwise it's tempting to finish an activity, and before you know it you've done too much. I've also used a timer for resting, to avoid the temptation to get up and carry on because I feel a bit better. If you have children who need something from you approximately every three-and-a-half minutes(!), it can be a useful way of explaining to them when you can or can't do something. Telling them that I can do the thing that they're asking me to when the timer goes off generally seems acceptable to them. If I don't set a timer, I usually don't get the rest that I planned.

STOPPING DISTANCE AND PRE-EMPTIVE BREAKS

The metaphor of a 'stopping distance' has been a useful pacing strategy for me. In practice this means stopping an activity when you're still feeling as though you could do more of it. Psychologically this can be incredibly challenging as the temptation to just do one more thing can be so great. Taking 'pre-emptive' or planned breaks rather than just breaks to recover from activity is a concept widely recommended in managing chronic illness. Taking scheduled breaks rather than reacting to symptoms is a proactive rather than reactive way of managing energy resources and can interrupt the boom/ bust cycle. Although not easy to do, taking scheduled rest can ultimately save you from doing too much and ultimately spending much longer being forced to rest. Pre-emptive rest works best if you schedule your rests around your day so that you have a plan and are more likely to avoid the 'just' trap. Ideally you should try to avoid draining your resources every day and aim to save some energy for healing rather than going overdrawn each day.

DON'T WAIT UNTIL THINGS ARE DONE TO REST!

Recently I noticed I was doing something which I thought was helping me but was actually draining my energy. I'd taken my boys to an hour-long tennis lesson and I found myself planning a list of things I could get done in that hour. When I got there all I wanted to do was sit and watch. I'd been trying to get ahead, but ahead of what, I wasn't sure! I realised that I often multi-task with the intention of getting ahead so that I can rest later. What usually happens though is that the time I save gets filled up with more tasks and I never actually reach that time when I can take a rest! That elusive time when you've got everything done will never happen.

ARMS AND LEGS

A particularly poignant memory from early on when I had Long Covid is struggling and failing to hang out some washing. I remember feeling devastated and hopeless that I couldn't do this apparently simple task and I drew all sorts of frightening conclusions about what this meant for me and my future. What I later discovered was that using my arms was sometimes more difficult and draining than using my legs. With POTS, my heart rate would shoot up with any activity, but doing something which looked simple, but involved both standing and using my arms at the same time, such as washing up at the sink, was just too challenging for my body at that time.

My point is that the apparent size of the task doesn't necessarily correlate with the demand it places on your body. It's easy to feel a sense of hopelessness when you feel that you can't 'even' do something which looks like a small thing. It doesn't necessarily mean that you'll never be able to do it. I now try to keep in mind that certain tasks are particularly demanding on me even when they don't look difficult to the outside world. I therefore need to account for these in my budget and try to balance them out with rest.

FIGURING OUT YOUR BEST TIMES

Working out the times in the day when you function best, whether that's physically, cognitively or emotionally, isn't straightforward and can change over time. When I struggled most with POTS, I would find that I was quite shaky in the mornings. However, a year later, if I have to do cognitive work which involves concentrating, it is better done in the morning when I seem to be able to think most clearly. If I try to exercise, such as doing a short Pilates class online, I'm better doing it later in the afternoon so that I don't risk running out of physical energy before I finish the day! Finding your own best patterns involves a lot of trial and error, flexibility and learning about yourself over time. Of course, when you do what isn't always within your control, particularly if you're trying to return to work. However, knowing your body and how it responds to particular tasks puts you in the best position to be able to organise what you can around your best times. This will not only benefit you but the people in your life who also need you to be at your best.

'CRITICAL LOW BATTERY'

As I switched on my laptop the other day, a 'critical low battery' alert popped up. As I immediately plugged it in, it occurred to me that I was being more responsive to the battery in my laptop than in my body, which I often take almost no notice of until the battery has run out! It would be so much easier to judge what we were capable of at any given time if we had a battery telling us what percentage energy we had left in our bodies. With Long Covid it's a constant challenge to work out what we can manage to do at any given time, but I do believe that our bodies are always giving us information about how we are, and what we need to do, as long as we pause long enough to tune in and listen. The signals that we're doing too much might start off quietly and be barely noticeable. For me they usually get increasingly louder until I listen. If I don't listen, I will be forced to stop later, but this can cost me more in the long run. Every time I do too much I'm reminded of the need to create the space to be quiet enough to listen and take notice of how I feel and what I'm capable of. For me this time is usually on my yoga mat or on a walk, but it could be any time or anything you do which creates the space in your day and your mind to listen to what your body is trying to say to you.

In this chapter I've summarised the things which have helped me the most with pacing myself. Before I end the chapter, I want to add one more thing. Pacing is really difficult! Perhaps there are people who don't find it as challenging not to overdo it as I do, but I'm yet to meet them. I once again come back to the idea of 'holding it lightly', which I feel can apply to most strategies I've explored. Pacing can be tedious and relentless and time and again I can be seduced by just wanting to get on with something which I know will be too much for my body. Sometimes I just want to lose myself a bit, and take a break from always thinking and working out what I'm capable of doing. Sometimes I just get fed up with having to think about it at all. At these times, despite everything I've said, I'll do something that's important to me and bear the consequences later. I figure that as long as I pace myself most of the time it allows me to push the boat out occasionally. If we can work to pace ourselves most, or even some, of the time then perhaps there can occasionally be room for playfulness and just letting go.

NOTES

Chapter Ten

Living 'Between'

'I'm still here, I'm still here.' It's late afternoon on one of those cold, bright autumnal days, a day like any other. I'm driving to pick up my son from school. For some reason, though, perhaps the sun catching the colours on the trees highlighting the changing of seasons, I'm taken somewhere else. For a moment, time is still, a mental snapshot of where I am right now. A moment of contentment, awe. How did I get here? I've walked my son to school, dealt with a broken washing machine, worked for a couple of hours, responded to emails and squeezed in 20 minutes of yoga. An extraordinary, ordinary day. Yet maybe I've rushed around too much, as I can feel that familiar drag of my body protesting. I'm okay, yet not okay. I'm both and neither. Perhaps I'm okay enough for now. Tomorrow will be more of the same, or different again. Not necessarily better or worse. Who knows?

This is not a story of recovery – not in the way that recovery is 'supposed' to go anyway. Long Covid was never going to play by the rules, to conform to the conventions of illness. If someone had told me 18 months ago that I wouldn't yet consider myself truly recovered, yet I'd be getting up early, navigating the frenzy that is getting my children out in time for school, going for a walk, doing the washing and writing,

I'd be over the moon but also confused. Wouldn't doing these things mean that I'd recovered?

I'm not entirely the person I was before catching Covid. The dictionary definition of recovery is 'a return to a normal state of health, mind, or strength' (*Oxford English Dictionary* 2021), and the verb 'recover' means to 'find again or obtain the return of something lost'. When I first got ill, I expected to be better within days, or at least weeks. I'd trawl through Facebook posts from people 'ahead' of me with similar symptoms, clinging on to claims of 10 or 12 weeks being the magic turning point where everything starts to improve. Thousands of us were doing it, comparing symptoms, swapping stories of 'week 10! It gets better at week 10!' followed by tales of relapse. Perhaps you were one of those people. Over and over again my hopes would be raised that finally I was starting to feel better, followed by the inevitable two or three steps backwards. We each counted days, then weeks, until eventually I stopped counting. I haven't returned to a 'normal' state of health or strength, and I haven't yet found all that I have lost. I've regained a lot, but pieces are still missing. If I do too much or try to exercise, it's as though my body goes into high alert mode until it restabilises itself. I budget, calculate, juggle and re-calculate my way through days, weeks and months. This gives me a quality of life that for a long time I didn't dare hope for. But I do miss those precious things which I could do without a second thought. I didn't know they were precious – I just didn't think about them.

LIVING 'BETWEEN' – NEITHER ILL NOR RECOVERED

In many ways, recovery is simple. You know exactly what recovery means, you can feel it in your body, and you just know when you're different, even if you can't entirely put it into words. It's simple, yet not straightforward. The most predictable thing about Long Covid is its unpredictability. Perhaps with any illness, progression is rarely as straightforward as it seems, and you just can't know until you're living it. Long Covid has left me in this strange no-man's land of not knowing where I fit, neither ill nor recovered, one foot in each camp, one side more than the other depending what day it is or what particular phase I'm going through. The further I'm able to venture into the 'real' world, the world of busy, high-functioning wellness, which was previously invisible to me, the more obvious my insufficiencies. In one moment, I can be both taken aback by how little I can do compared to my pre-Covid self, yet also how much I can do compared to my 'ill' self. Occasionally I catch myself doing something which, if someone else saw, they would find it hard to believe that I hadn't entirely recovered. You might see someone with Long Covid doing anything within certain limits, but what you won't see is the 'payback': the rest of the day or week in bed because they blew the day's budget doing the food shopping or going for a walk. They might also be living 'between'.

When we think and talk about recovery, we often focus on the physical. When you're so incapacitated and feeling so ill, it's hard to think of anything else beyond regaining your physical health and abilities. But on emerging from the relentlessness of symptoms, it is hard not to find yourself changed in other ways. Although many of my symptoms have subsided, my sense is not of a return to a previous state, but of travelling further down a road which winds ahead into the distance, an unknown future.

Perhaps we need a fuller definition of recovery, or to define our own. Perhaps recovery is in the personal, a process of finding ways to go forward in life and engage with the world in the ways which matter most to you. Perhaps it isn't in the word we use; it is what it means to us and how Long Covid positions us – or how we can position it – in our lives. For me it's about recovery of trust in my body, or a small reminder or discovery of who I am beyond Long Covid. Sometimes, it's just about getting through the day. An idea of recovery as a linear process or a return from illness back to wellness implies always moving and progressing. It allows little room for wandering paths or standing still for a while. Yet when we go through something as huge as this, standing still long enough to look around and catch up with ourselves might have some value. Standing still has little place in a culture of progression, business and reaching goals, yet when we move too quickly, we can lose connection with what matters most to us. I've always viewed recurrences of symptoms, or new symptoms, as relapses or backward steps, yet when I've been able to see a broader picture, often only with the benefit of time, they also look like moments of pause; times when my body has reminded me that I'm trying to go too fast. Holding on too tightly to linear progress and recovery may obscure other things of value.

Jo Bowlby, in her conversation with Fearne Cotton on her podcast Happy Place (Cotton 2021) reminds us that we cannot always analyse our way through things with the rational mind. She refers to the intellectual mind, the emotional mind, the heart mind, the soul mind and the spiritual mind. The soul mind is the imagination, a sense of stillness. 'We have to start embracing stillness again...it's not just the yin to the yang of doing...being and doing...it is also that place where our imagination opens up, it's where the magic comes in again.'

DO WE GAIN OR GROW FROM
SUFFERING TRAUMA?

I haven't given up hoping that my body will feel 'normal' again. I would always choose for Long Covid to never have happened to me. Yet there is something that, dare I say it, I've gained, that now I wouldn't want to lose. As human beings, we seek to make meaning of our experiences and want to believe that difficult times bring reward. 'Post-traumatic growth' (Tedeschi and Calhoun 1996) is the concept that people can gain new understandings of the world, themselves, their relationships and how they want to live their lives following a traumatic incident or period in their lives. I'm reminded of the Japanese art of Kintsugi, where broken pottery is repaired using lacquer dusted with powdered gold or silver. Rather than being something to disguise, the breakage and repair of an object is seen as part of its history. Not only that, but the repairs are purposely illuminated. Kirsten Weir, in 'Life after COVID-19: Making space for growth' (2020) used this as a metaphor for emerging stronger from trauma. While I yearn for my body to return to its original, uncracked form, perhaps there is something in the value of what emerges from times of trauma that can also be true.

But does trauma inevitably lead to us growing or gaining in some way, or is this just a way of bringing positivity to a dire situation? On Elizabeth Day's podcast 'How to Fail' (2021), presenter and actor Graham Norton describes the effects of his own near-death experience, when he was stabbed at the age of 25. He tells of a burst of feeling he experienced on recovery, as though he could do anything and 'knew the importance of everything'. This didn't last long, but what stayed with him was a sense that 'I'm alive...I win...it set me up for the rest of my life…it gave me a really good attitude to risk, and to failure…it was a very useful and powerful life lesson at that time'.

Recently in *The New Yorker*, Meghan O'Gieblyn asks whether there are hidden advantages to pain and suffering (2021). She states, 'the events we consider most central to our identities are often tragedies – an illness survived, an addiction tamed…as though we believed adversity to be the price of wisdom and personal improvement'. She also writes about Paul Bloom's book, *The Sweet Spot: The Pleasures of Suffering and the Search for Meaning* (2021), where he explores the relationship between suffering, meaning and happiness, finding evidence to suggest that happiness and meaning are correlated, and that we may even seek out pain with the expected reward of pleasure or meaning. However, he suggests that when suffering is not chosen or within our control in some way, the reward of meaning may be absent. O'Gieblyn concludes that although we may not be able to avoid pain, we can have some say in the sense we make of it and the narratives we build around it.

I know that I am different. In recent weeks and months, I've had a sense of settling in to the person I was always supposed to be but was held back by…I'm not sure what – going through the motions of ordinary life? Convention? Whatever it was, I think I'm a little bit more 'me'. Long Covid has shifted my sense of where I fit and what I want to do with my time. Some of these changes are small, but not insignificant. I've uncovered parts of myself that perhaps were always there but obscured by layers of unquestioned ideas about how to be. I feel more daring, yet I also have a new enjoyment for what used to look like the boring and ordinary. I get a ridiculous amount of pleasure from taking myself off for a walk, and I'm grateful for an uneventful day. Now when I go to bed, I rarely question whether I'll wake up – I've almost forgotten what that felt like. When I do remember, it's easier to find perspective. I think I have a new sensitivity and emotionality for other peoples' stories. Most significantly my relationship with risk is altered. I still get stressed by day-to-day challenges, often the trivial, but this is against a backdrop of life also being a playful adventure, where it matters less if things work out or not. There's a new freedom in knowing that, in the end, it doesn't really matter. Perhaps this will fade over time, but, like Graham Norton, I can't imagine returning entirely to how I was before. I'm more myself than I've ever felt before, yet I'd still choose for Long Covid never to have happened to me – both things are true.

This isn't an argument for positivity. Long Covid is a truly horrendous experience, with daily reminders of what has been lost. It's also not the whole story. There's a lot about it that can't be changed, but sometimes I do have some say in what I do next. I don't know whether the good outweighs the bad; whether the nebulous idea of growth is compensation for pain. I often feel not. But as O'Gieblyn suggests, we don't find meaning in a cost–benefit analysis approach to life. Life is not a scorecard, but a story (O'Gieblyn 2021).

IS ACCEPTANCE IMPORTANT?

Recovery is complex, multi-faceted and individual, but where does that leave you when Long Covid is still there, every day, in your life? Even in respect of purely physical recovery, it is too early to know how Long Covid will play out on a global and individual level. Should we be trying to accept it some-how? A study of acceptance in chronic illness by Mazurek and Lurbiecki (2014) suggests that 'the greater the acceptance of disease is, the less mental discomfort and less severe negative emotions there are'. The concept of acceptance came from psychiatrist Kubler-Ross' work with people with terminal illness (Kubler-Ross and Kessler 2005), the acceptance of a new reality being the final stage of grief, although this theory has been criticised and often oversimplified as it has been absorbed into popular culture. Acceptance is often held up as something to achieve, as though it is a fixed state to reach, which risks leaving people feeling that they're coming up short by failing to accept a new reality. For me, acceptance of Long Covid feels too close to letting go or giving in. It would feel like drawing it closer, which is the last thing I want to do. I fear that acceptance would separate me from the precious energy that I need to stand up to it, and to keep doing the things I need to do to get me through. Perhaps my struggle with acceptance is bound up with anger. Anger gets a bad press because it can be used destructively, but it also speaks to what I care about and fuels my energy to keep getting through the day and prioritising what matters most.

Despite the apparent value of anger as fuel for action, I don't wish to spend my time in a constant state of battle and trying to get the upper hand over Long Covid. This would mean living my life always in relation to it. Metaphors around fighting and battling have been absorbed into the language of illness – the inference being that we are 'supposed' to fight it, to not let it win. Yet when I've managed to let go a little, to loosen ever so slightly the reins of control over Long Covid, I get closer to a quieter way of being, a state which suggests that my nervous system is in parasympathetic, healing mode, which brings with it a feeling of relief and peace, however fleeting.

For now, Long Covid is a part of my life. I don't want a battle; nor am I ready to accept it. Perhaps a middle ground can be found, where it doesn't dominate everything but I'm not denying it in ways which could make it worse. I acknowledge its presence for now, but I don't accept it. Accommodating it would feel too much like giving it a permanent home. For now, it can have its place alongside me, having its say in certain parts of my life, but not in everything. This might just sound like a matter of language, but the language we use shapes our experience and how we respond. Long Covid isn't me, it is part of my life for now. Sometimes it gets to decide what I can or can't do; other times I have more say. Long Covid is not the whole of who I am. It doesn't say anything about me other than how I manage it.

What might acknowledging Long Covid look like in practice? It might mean riding out a symptom because you know you've got through it before. You might remember the small thing which helped last time. It could mean making a medical appointment, asking other people with Long Covid about a particular issue or doing something to calm your nervous system. Long Covid sometimes still frightens me, but I usually have some ideas about what I could do next. I might not be able to go for a walk today, but I could do breathing exercises, yoga or just be still and listen to what my body needs. Sometimes it means adapting plans and deciding what to let go of. Other days I can do what I want to do despite it. I can still take some action even when I can't be active.

I find myself wanting to somehow wrap this book up neatly; to draw some kind of conclusions which make some sense out of everything. But this is not an endpoint, or the end of the story, just a snapshot in time. Recovery isn't a finite, solely physical experience with a clear end point, but an individual, complex process evolving in real time. When we divide illness or recovery into the physical and the psychological, we miss so much of the complexity of how we function and how we might be helped and help ourselves to feel better.

I hope that by the time you're reading this we know a lot more about Long Covid and how it can be treated. I hope that Long Covid will be taken seriously as a risk of having even a mild Covid infection, and I hope that research and discussion in relation to Long Covid will have an impact on how people with chronic pain or poorly understood illnesses are seen and treated. This is an opportunity to change the narratives about symptoms and illnesses which don't necessarily show up on traditional medical tests.

This book is about breaking free from the effects of Long Covid, but this is not a once-and-for-all process, but a practice of untethering, loosening the binds bit by bit, reclaiming the parts of your life which matter to you most and trusting your own sense of what to do at any particular time. It happens in the small actions we take every day. There is no map of recovery from people who have gone before us. We are pioneers, figuring it out for ourselves, between ourselves, and it's what we've done every day.

I hope that in this book you have felt moments of recognition which relate to your own struggles and experiences, and that you've found something which gets you through a particularly bad moment. This book isn't about one right way of doing things; it is one person's story which I hope will contribute to a much wider conversation about what helps. This is just one set of ideas, but the more knowledges we generate, the more options we have for going forward. I would love to hear your thoughts and ideas. With Long Covid, the view looks different every day. One day you might feel positive change, the next, a seemingly backwards step or an overwhelming grief for what has been lost. All of these might happen within a single day. We do not have to choose between being okay and not okay. We do not have to be defined by one single story, or one set of ideas about how to be. Recovery is a process, not a completion. This is not the end, but in the words of Lucille Clifton in her poem 'i am not done yet' (1987), 'less certain than I seem, more certain than I was...I continue to continue'.

FOR REFLECTION

- In what ways are you different as a result of Long Covid? Are any of these changes or differences welcome? In what ways?
- What have you gained from your experience that you didn't have before? Have you uncovered anything that wasn't visible to you?
- What else do you need to recover, other than the physical?
- What would you like to move towards?
- What steps could you take to move in this direction?

NOTES

Team of Life – Creating Your Own Team Sheet

The following questions are designed to get you thinking about your own team. You can alter them according to the sport or alternative metaphor you choose to use. The questions are orientated towards considering your life as a whole, but you might want to think about them particularly in the context of the people who would be in your 'Long Covid team'. There's space to note your initial responses below each question, but I'd encourage you to find somewhere where you can write more extensively in order to include everything that comes into your head.

I. **Goalkeeper, Safety, Centre** – Who can be relied on to look out for you? (maybe a person, group or organisation)

2. **Defence** – Who else helps you to protect what is precious and important to you?

3. **Coach** – Who teaches you or has taught you the most important things you've learned so far in life? What are some of the things they have taught you?

4. **Offence/Attack** – Who encourages and helps you to score?

5. **Other teammates** – Who are your teammates in life? Whose company do you enjoy?

6. **Your position** – Where would you place yourself on this team?

_____

_____

_____

_____

7. **Substitutes** – Are there some people who help you at certain times and not others? When are they helpful/not helpful? How have you learned the difference?

_____

_____

_____

_____

8. **Spectators, fans, supporters in the stands** – Who are the people hoping you do well? (living or non-living)

_____

_____

_____

_____

9. **Key values you're defending** – What are some of the key values you're defending in your team? What is the team standing for? What are your goals that they are defending?

_____

_____

_____

_____

10. **Home ground** – Where do you feel most at home? (this could be more than one place, somewhere you visit regularly or used to go or it could be in your imagination)

_____

_____

_____

_____

11. **Team song** – Is there a song that means a lot to you at the moment? Why is it significant?

_____

_____

_____

_____

12. **First aid kit** – What supports your team when things get difficult? What's in your first aid kit?

_____

_____

_____

_____

This metaphor can be expanded and elaborated on. Denborough (2014) suggests other themes to explore such as team emblem, motto, mascot, sponsor and manager. He extends the metaphor further, describing parts two, three and four of the exercise. These include creating a 'goal map', celebrating the goal you've already achieved and looking forward to the next goals, considering the training you will do and the adversities you might face. For more information, see Denborough (2014, pp.96–106).

References

Beddington, E. (2021) 'The seven types of rest: I spent a week trying them all. Could they help end my exhaustion?' *The Guardian*, 25 November. Available at www.theguardian.com/lifeandstyle/2021/nov/25/the-seven-types-of-rest-i-spent-a-week-trying-them-all-could-they-help-end-my-exhaustion. Accessed 15.12.21.

Bloom, P. (2021) *The Sweet Spot: The Pleasures of Suffering and the Search for Meaning.* New York: Echo Press.

Broyard, A. (1993) *Intoxicated by My Illness: And Other Writings on Life and Death.* New York: Fawcett Columbine.

Clifton, L. (1987) 'i am not done yet.' Published in *The Collected Poems of Lucille Clifton 1965–2010.* New York: BOA Editions Ltd.

Cotton, F. (Host) (2021, November 15) Happy Place: Jo Bowlby. [Audio podcast episode]. In *Happy Place.* Accessed 29.12.21.

Dani, M., Dirksen, D., Taraborrelli, P., Torocastro, M., Panagopoulas, D., Sutton, R. & Boon Lim, P. (2021) 'Autonomic dysfunction in "long COVID": Rationale, physiology and management strategies.' *Clinical Medicine* 21, 1, e63–e67.

Day, E. (Host). (2021, May 26). How to Fail: Graham Norton. S II, Ep I. [Audio podcast episode]. In *How To Fail With Elizabeth Day.* Accessed 19.12.21.

Day, E. (2021) Elizabeth Day: 'This is why I got a tattoo'. *You Magazine,* September 12. Available at https://www.you.co.uk/elizabeth-day-this-is-why-I-got-a-tattoo-/# Accessed 18.12.21.

Denborough, D. (2008) *Collective Narrative Practice: Responding to Individuals, Groups, and Communities Who Have Experienced Trauma.* Adelaide, Australia: Dulwich Centre Publications.

Denborough, D. (2014) *Retelling the Stories of Our Lives: Everyday Narrative Therapy to Draw Inspiration and Transform Experience.* New York: W.W. Norton & Company, Inc.

Eccleston, C. & Crombez, C. (1999) 'Pain demands attention: A cognitive active model of the interruptive function of pain.' *Psychological Bulletin 125*, 3, 356–366.

Frank, A.W. (1995) *The Wounded Storyteller: Body, Illness, and Ethics.* Chicago, IL: University of Chicago Press.

Garner, P. (2020) 'Covid-19 and fatigue – a game of snakes and ladders.' *The BMJ Opinion* 19 May. Available at https://blogs.bmj.com/bmj/2020/05/19/paul-garner-covid-19-and-fatigue-a-game-of-snakes-and-ladders. Accessed 17.12.21.

George, J. (2021) *A Still Life: A Memoir.* [Online], London: Bloomsbury Publishing Plc.

Gergen, K. (1994) *Realities and Relationships; Soundings in Social Construction.* Cambridge, MA: Harvard University Press.

Gilbert, E. (2016) *Big Magic.* London: Bloomsbury.

Greenspan, N. (2020) *COVID Rehab & Recovery Series: All About That Breath!* Lecture 21, July 5. [Video]. Available at https://pulmonary-wellness.org/pulmonary-wellness-lecture-series-2020. Accessed 26.12.21.

Habib, N. (2019) *Activate Your Vagus Nerve: Unleash Your Body's Natural Ability to Heal.* Berkeley, CA: Ulysses Press.

Hare, D. (dir.) (2021) *Beat the Devil.* [Film] Sky Arts, 11.11.21.

Hof, W. (2020) *The Wim Hof Method: Activate Your Potential, Transcend Your Limits.* London: Rider.

The Holistic Psychologist [the.holistic.psychologist] (2021, June 29). Boundaries Around Urgency Culture Sound like: Instagram. Instagram.com/the.holistic.psychologist.

Kubler-Ross, E. & Kessler, D. (2005) *On Grief and Grieving: Finding the Meaning of Grief through the Five Stages of Loss.* New York: Scribner.

May, K. (2020) *Wintering: The Power of Rest and Retreat in Difficult Times.* London: Rider.

Mazurek, J. & Lurbiecki, J. (2014) 'Acceptance of illness scale and its clinical impact.' Available at PubMed.gov, https://pubmed.ncbi. nlm.nih.gov/24720106. Accessed 19.12.21.

National Institute for Health and Care Excellence (NICE) (2021) Myalgic encephalomyelitis (or encephalopathy)/chronic fatigue syndrome: Diagnosis and management. NG206. 29 October.

Nestor, J. (2021) *Breath: The New Science of a Lost Art.* London: Penguin Life.

Newsnight (2021) BBC2, 19 July.

Newson, L., Lewis, R. & O'Hara, M. (2021) 'Long Covid and menopause – the important role of hormones in Long Covid must be considered.' *Maturitas 152,* 74.

O'Gieblyn, M. (2021) 'Are there hidden advantages to pain and suffering?' *The New Yorker,* 8 November. Available at www.newyorker. com/magazine/2021/11/15/are-there-hidden-advantages-to-pain-and-suffering-hurts-so-good-leigh-cowart-the-sweet-spot-paul-bloom/amp. Accessed 19.12.21.

OneWelbeck (2021) *Dr Boon Lin in conversation with his patient Natalie, discussing Long Covid recovery.* [Video]. Available at https://m.youtube.com/watch?v=KoktH5CXy21. Accessed 17.12.21.

Oxford English Dictionary (n.d.) Recovery. Available at https://www. oed.com. Accessed 17.12.21

Panorama (2021) BBC1, Season 30, episode 24. 12 July 2021.

PoTS UK (2020) 'Medication: Medication.' Available at www.potsuk. org/managingpots/medication-2. Accessed 08.03.22.

Ramey, S. (2020) *The Lady's Handbook for her Mysterious Illness.* [Online]. London: Fleet.

Risen, C. (2021) 'Mihaly Csikszentmihalyi, the father of "Flow", dies at 87.' *The New York Times,* 27 October. Available at www.nytimes. com/2021/10/27/science/mihaly-csikszentmihalyi-dead.amp. html. Accessed 20.12.21.

Roos, S. (2002) *Chronic Sorrow: A Living Loss.* New York: Brunner-Routledge.

RUN-DMC/Gez Medinger (2020, November 24) *Here's How You Treat Long Covid – Lessons from MCAS – Dr Tina Peers.* [Video].https://m. youtube.com/watch?v=slCDOKn6pR4. Accessed 18.12.21.

Stewart, S. *et al.* (2021) 'Long COVID risk – a signal to address sex hormones and women's health.' *The Lancet 11*, 100242. Available at https://www.thelancet.com/journals/lanepe/article/PIIS2666-7762(21)00228-3/fulltext. Accessed 14.02.22.

Tang, A. (2021) cited in Hopper, J. 'Embracing dark skies.' *Planet Mindful 20*, Nov/Dec, p.37.

Tedeschi, R.G. & Calhoun, L.G. (1996) 'The Posttraumatic Growth Inventory: Measuring the positive legacy of trauma.' *Journal of Traumatic Stress 9*, 3, 455–472. https://doi.org/10.1002/jts.2490090305.

Wallston, K. (2001) 'Control beliefs: Health perspectives.' *International Encyclopedia of the Social & Behavioral Sciences*, 2724–2726. Available at www.sciencedirect.com/science/article/pii/B0080430767037992. Accessed 19.12.21.

Weingarten, K. (2001) 'Making sense of illness narratives: Braiding theory, practice and the embodied life.' *Dulwich Centre Publications*. Available at https://dulwichcentre.com.au/articles-J-narrative-therapy/illness-narratives. Accessed 18.12.21.

Weingarten, K. (2013a) 'The "cruel radiance of what is": Helping couples live with chronic illness.' *Family Process 52*, 83–101, 96.

Weingarten, K. (2013b) 'Understanding families struggling daily with the effects of health problems.' Available at https://dulwichcentre.com.au/understanding-families-struggling-daily-with-the-effects-of-health-problems. Accessed 18.12.21.

Weinstock, L.B. *et al.* (2021) 'Mast cell activation symptoms are prevalent in Long-COVID.' *International Journal of Infectious Disease*, Nov, 112, 217–226.

Weir, K. (2020) 'Life after COVID-19: Making space for growth.' *American Psychological Association*. Available at www.apa.org/monitor/2020/06/covid-life-after. Accessed 19.12.21.

White, M. (2006) 'Working with People Who Are Suffering the Consequences of Multiple Trauma: A Narrative Perspective.' In D. Denborough (ed.), *Trauma: Narrative Responses to Traumatic Experience*. Adelaide, Australia: Dulwich Centre Publications.

Yoga for Long Covid with Suzy Bolt 360mindbodysoul (2021, July 7). *Interview by Suzy Bolt with Dr Tanya Patrick and Dr Claire*

Phipps. [Video]. YouTube. https://m.youtube.com/watch?v=
K6ny8pgXZMA. Accessed 18.12.21.

Yoga With Adriene (2021) [YouTube channel]. YouTube. https://m.
youtube.com/channel/UCFKE7WVJfvaHW5q283SxchA. Accessed
15.12.21.

Resources

BOOKS

Denborough, D. (2014) *Retelling the Stories of Our Lives: Everyday Narrative Therapy to Draw Inspiration and Transform Experience.* New York: W.W. Norton & Company, Inc.

George, J. (2021) *A Still Life: A Memoir.* London: Bloomsbury Publishing Plc.

Habib, N. (2019) *Activate Your Vagus Nerve: Unleash Your Body's Natural Ability to Heal.* Berkeley, CA: Ulysses Press.

Hof, W. (2020) *The Wim Hof Method: Activate Your Potential, Transcend Your Limits.* London: Rider.

May, K. (2020) *Wintering: The Power of Rest and Retreat in Difficult Times.* London: Rider.

Nestor, J. (2021) *Breath: The New Science of a Lost Art.* London: Penguin Life.

Weingarten, K. (2001) 'Making sense of illness narratives: Braiding theory, practice and the embodied life'. Dulwich Centre Publications. Available at https://dulwichcentre.com.au/articles-J-narrative-therapy/illness-narratives. Accessed 18.12.21.

WEBSITES

Dysautonomia International: www.dysautonomiainternational.org
The Holistic Psychologist: https://instagram.com/the.holistic. psychologist
Long Covid Physio: https://longcovid.physio
Lottie Murphy Pilates: www.lottiemurphy.com
PoTS UK: https://www.potsuk.org.
Pulmonary Wellness Foundation: pulmonarywellness.org
Stasis Post-Covid Online Programme: https://www.stasis.life
Yoga with Adriene – YouTube: https://m.youtube.com/user/yoga withadriene

APPS

Balance
Breethe
Wattson Blue App

Subject Index

Author Index